QUANTUM INTEGRATIVE MEDICINE

Also by
AMIT GOSWAMI, PH.D.

The Self-Aware Universe
Science and Spirituality
The Visionary Window
Physics of the Soul
The Quantum Doctor
God Is Not Dead
Creative Evolution
How Quantum Activism Can Save Civilization
Quantum Creativity
Quantum Economics
The Everything Answer Book
Quantum Politics
Quantum Activation: Changing Obstacles into Opportunities (with Carl David Blake and Gary Stuart)
See the World as a Five Layered Cake

Also by
AMIT GOSWAMI, PH.D. & VALENTINA R. ONISOR, M.D.

Quantum Spirituality
The Quantum Brain

QUANTUM INTEGRATIVE MEDICINE

A NEW PARADIGM for
HEALTH, DISEASE PREVENTION,
and HEALING

**AMIT GOSWAMI, PH.D.
& VALENTINA R. ONISOR, M.D.**

Monkfish Book Publishing Company
Rhinebeck, New York

Quantum Integrative Medicine: A New Paradigm for Health, Disease Prevention, and Healing © Copyright 2023 by Amit Goswami, Ph.D and Valentina R. Onisor, M.D.

All rights reserved. No part of this book may be used or reproduced in any manner without the consent of the publisher except in critical articles or reviews. Contact the publisher for information.

Paperback ISBN 978-1-948626-87-3
eBook ISBN 978-1-948626-88-0

Library of Congress Cataloging-in-Publication Data

Names: Goswami, Amit, author. | Onisor, Valentina R., author.
Title: Quantum integrative medicine : a new paradigm for health, disease prevention, and healing / Amit Goswami, PH.D & Valentina R. Onisor, M.D.
Description: Rhinebeck, NY : Monkfish Book Publishing Company, [2023] | Includes bibliographical references and index.
Identifiers: LCCN 2022043029 (print) | LCCN 2022043030 (ebook) | ISBN 9781948626873 (paperback) | ISBN 9781948626880 (eBook)
Subjects: LCSH: Integrative medicine. | Holistic medicine.
Classification: LCC R733 .G676 2023 (print) | LCC R733 (ebook) | DDC 610--dc23/eng/20221025
LC record available at https://lccn.loc.gov/2022043029
LC ebook record available at https://lccn.loc.gov/2022043030

Monkfish Book Publishing Company
22 East Market Street, Suite 304
Rhinebeck, NY 12572
(845) 876-4861
monkfishpublishing.com

*This book is dedicated to all interested users,
to all medical students who will practice integrative
medicine in their profession, and to all researchers
who will take the paradigm further.*

CONTENTS

Preface ix
Introduction: The Time Is Ripe for Quantum Integrative Medicine 1

PART 1: A NEW PERSPECTIVE FOR THE SCIENCE OF MEDICINE

1. Hardware and Software: Why We Need to Include More Than the Material Body for Healthcare and Quantum Integrative Medicine to Work 27
2. Know Thy Self, Oh, Quantum Doctor 51
3. Prevention: A New and Essential Perspective 65
4. Resonance: The Secret of Being Positive—and the Expanded Consciousness, Wellness, and Happiness That Come with It 76
5. Who Is a Healer? 89

PART 2: THE QUANTUM SCIENCE OF HOLISTIC HEALTH AND PREVENTIVE MEDICINE

6. Vital Body Medicine: General Principles, Acupuncture, and Homeopathy 105
7. Comparative Medicine: Integrating Ayurveda and Traditional Chinese Medicine 123

8. Preventive Medicine Lesson 1: Body Types and Corresponding Lifestyles 141
9. Preventive Medicine Lesson 2: The Quantum Science of the Chakras 155
10. Quantum Mind: Meaning, Emotions, and Medicine 165
11. Quantum Science of the Heart Chakra and Women's Breast Cancer 181
12. Preventive Medicine Lesson 3: How to Deal with Mentalization 192

PART 3: UNLEASHING THE FULL POWER OF QUANTUM INTEGRATIVE MEDICINE

13. Preventive Medicine Lesson 4: Nutrition 199
14. Preventive Medicine Lesson 5: Quantum Yoga for Quantum Healing 231
15. Preventive Medicine Lesson 6: Going Deep in Your Practice for Quantum Healing 241
16. Quantum Gerontology: Live Quantum, Live Healthy, Live Longer, Die Happy 250
17. Preventive Medicine Lesson 7: Holistic Health, Quantum Style 276

Bibliography 283
Index 291
About the Authors 307

PREFACE

I (Amit) have been working on health and healing since 1999, after being inspired by Dalai Lama to apply the integrative ideas of quantum science to practical everyday problems in people's lives. My book, *The Quantum Doctor*, published in 2004, resulted from my initial efforts.

The science of medicine, as we see it, has two major problems. The first and foremost is that there are several disparate medicine systems based on different health paradigms. Modern allopathic medicine based on the primacy of matter (the material body is all there is for us) and, in particular, molecular biology (biology is the chemistry of molecules), which works in certain compartments of disease such as those caused by bacteria and viruses but is relatively ineffective for chronic diseases and has dangerous side effects; also, in the aftermath of cure by allopathy when the physical symptoms are gone but patients are still suffering.

For chronic disease, age-old traditional medicine systems developed in India (Ayurveda) and China (Traditional Chinese Medicine) millennia ago, along with a relatively modern medicine system called homeopathy, work much better and without side effects. Collectively, these and other ancient traditional medicine systems are called Alternative (or Complementary) medicine systems and their health paradigm includes nonmaterial concepts of vital and mental bodies in addition to the physical.

Second, modern allopathic medicine is mostly evidence-based. In physics, which is the fundamental basis of all science in the materialist worldview, a proper paradigm of science requires both theory and evidence. In other words, evidence-based science is bound to be incomplete and inconsistent.

The alternative medicine systems have theories but they are based on an ancient dualistic worldview (such as mind and matter being separate entities), which leaves unsolved the embarrassing question of how these separate entities, having nothing in common, interact.

Quantum physics gives us the needed integrative metaphysics—consciousness is the ground of all being in which matter and the mind are quantum possibilities for consciousness to choose from.

My first task was to use the new quantum metaphysics to provide a basic science for the systems of alternative medicine and thus begin a tentative integration of medicine. This was accomplished in *The Quantum Doctor*.

What was still lacking, though, was a unified theory of health and for the development of a science of medicine as a science of health used to treat disease as a health disorder. If we discover such a theory, then obviously, we should be able to prevent disease in the first place.

Much more expertise in specifics was needed for such an endeavour. In 2016, Valentina Onisor, M.D., trained in both allopathic and most systems of alternative medicine as well—Ayurveda, yoga, naturopathy, aromatherapy, and homeopathy—joined hands with me. Valentina has also been looking for an integrative medicine since her student days. We have been researching the development of an integrative medicine based on quantum science ever since.

This book is the culmination of our efforts and represents a union of our voices. We think we have succeeded. Much further research will be needed of course to verify the details, but the basics of the approach have already been verified by empirical data.

Who is our audience? We intend this book to be useful to both laypeople on the consumer side of medicine and professionals on the delivery side. Moreover, we want this book to serve masters and Ph.D.

students at our own educational enterprise under the auspices of the Department of Quantum Science of Health, Prosperity, and Happiness, at the University of Technology in Jaipur, India; this facility is fully affiliated with the Government of India.

It has been a difficult task to find a writing style suitable for multiple audiences. Eventually, we decided to employ a user-friendly style, no apologies. In that spirit, we present the material in the first person throughout most of the book, but please be aware: Every paragraph has been coauthored by both of us.

We also wish to thank Atish Mozumder, Ph.D., and Krishanu Goswami for their careful critique of the manuscript in its early stages.

—AMIT GOSWAMI AND VALENTINA R. ONISOR

Introduction

THE TIME IS RIPE FOR QUANTUM INTEGRATIVE MEDICINE

Post materialists, including avant-garde medical doctors, usually talk about integrative medicine in the context of the holistic health of our body. There is now some acceptance of the idea that mind matters and that love matters in our consideration of health and healing. But of course, there is no viable new theory of the mind or of love that is different from what materialists think of as mind. Love, the emotions, etc., are epiphenomena of matter and are considered to have no role to play.

However, several new discoveries demand that we develop a new approach to how we deal with health and healing:

1. The most crucial discovery has come from quantum physics: Consciousness is the ground of all being, of all our experiences. All science must be based on the primacy of consciousness. Why is this important? Modern allopathic medicine is mechanical, totally objective. Even in holistic extensions of modern medicine, people try to maintain objectivity. The quantum worldview is saying this is a myopic view. You count, and your doctor's subjectivity counts too, in matters of health and healing.
2. Besides our biochemical body, we have a bioelectric body, at the skin, which is sensitive to our feelings. In this way, measurements

of this biofield enable us to measure feelings. Our experiences of feelings, though subjective, are real and even measurable albeit indirectly. These measurements are demonstrating the scientific viability of the idea that we have a nonphysical vital body associated with physical.
3. In a similar vein, functional magnetic resonance imaging (fMRI) technique allows us to measure changes in the brain as we change our thinking. Our experiences of thought are also measurable and real even though mind is nonphysical.
4. Lifestyle matters to our health as much as or even more than the diseases that we catch through injuries and bacteria and viruses even when we practice good hygiene. In particular, negative emotional stress causes various chronic diseases; in contrast, positive emotions, meaning, and purpose leads to health and improves longevity.
5. Our physiology—organ functions—are not genetic in origin; instead, they are epigenetic, their origin is outside of the genes. Their source is nonlocal, and therefore, nonmaterial. Why is this important? Because human physiology is not a permanent fixture but is changeable via creativity.
6. We have little brains in the body areas of the heart as well as of the navel. In quantum science this means there is self-identity in these areas of the body. Your creative experiences of feeling in these areas are positive, such as self-worth (at the navel) and love (at the heart). Your positivity is supremely important for health and healing.

Responding to this welcome development in empirical data, the research reported in this book has produced a highly needed theory of human health and healing. A crucial ingredient of this theory is a science of feelings and emotions incorporating the idea of feeling centers, located not only the brain but also in the body, called chakras.

With both prongs—theory and experiment—of the science of

health and healing at hand, we have finally been able to achieve a complete integration of conventional and alternative medicine, an effort that began with the publication of Amit's book *The Quantum Doctor* in 2004.

In the absence of a theory of health, conventional medicine has been largely forced to stay disease-centered. Only when you have a disease can clinical studies develop drugs or surgery (or radiation in the case of cancer) and your allopathic physician treat you to alleviate your symptoms. Limited prevention guidance can be given on the basis of improved diagnostic procedures, to be sure; however, even this guidance only covers physical symptoms and your physical body. How about the rest of you?

Alternative medicine—Ayurveda and Traditional Chinese Medicine—are preventive in spirit, but their efforts are limited because of the incomplete nature of the theories of these traditions.

We declare that the integration achieved here—Quantum Integrative Medicine—is a bona fide preventive medicine. We have succeeded in providing you with the most avant-garde techniques of nutrition of all five of our bodies—physical, vital, mental, soul (supramental), and spirit—to give you a reliable handle for disease prevention.

The most important theoretical development of this preventive integration of medicine is this: It is our contention that an elevated physiology for organs in the navel and the heart areas has been universally available for all humanity for millennia. This higher physiology has kept us away from chronic disease like cancer. All this is rapidly changing today because of faulty worldview and lifestyle. The physiology that conventional medicine assumes is not right to this extent and human physiology is not a given and unchangeable one either. We have rediscovered the mechanism of changing the physiology of organs in some scientific practical detail. It is called vital creativity.

You may even be a little squeamish about mental creativity when it comes to inner development. Can you engage in vital creativity, inner development in the vital area? Item 6, above, shows that you have several selves in your body. You were familiar with having experiences in the navel and the heart when you were a child, but the materialist culture kept you away from those experiences by denigrating feelings, especially feelings in the body. Reclaim them. We will show you how. Then, vital creativity will no longer seem difficult.

ELABORATION

Mainstream medicine practice—modern medicine or allopathy—is based on the philosophy of material monism—primacy of matter. So the import of the message from quantum physics is as unambiguous as it is timely: A radical revision of modern medicine is called for. The health-care crisis that we see today demands immediate action to achieve this paradigm shift.

Items 2, 3, and 4, above, point out some areas where change is most needed. We all know that besides our sensory experiences of the material world, we also have experiences of emotions—thoughts mixed with feelings, pure thoughts, and, for some people, even pure feelings. These experiences certainly affect our sense of well-being: We feel stressed out with negative emotions; likewise, we feel elated and expanded when we are able to emote positively.

Now that we know that our lifestyle matters to our health, that a lifestyle in which negative emotional stress dominates means illness and one in which positive emotions dominate means wellness, wouldn't it be nice to have a health science that takes account of these experiences as well, now that we know that they are measurable? What we feel is energy, traditionally called *prana* in India, where this energy's existence was first officially noted; *chi* in China, where it was also extensively studied; and vital energy in English. Vital energy is a measurable quantity.

In *The Quantum Doctor*, I (Amit) discussed Kirlian photography being used for measurement of the biofield associated with our feelings. Additionally, we now also have the research of Dr. Masaru Emoto on water, showing how using various emotional words (spoken or even just thought) affects the formation of water crystals. Even though he was very much criticized for his lack of research methodology and a credible theory, Dr. Emoto's experiments, which have been replicated by another highly credible researcher, Dean Radin, clearly show that the crystallization of water can be influenced by human emotions.

Even more definitive is the evidence of coherent biophoton emission by the dynamic biofield of a person of awakened heart by psychologist Gioacchino Pagliaro.

What do we think? The objects of thought convey meaning, and the fMRI (functional magnetic resonance imaging technique) data demonstrates that this too is measurable (we detail this in our book *The Quantum Brain*). To have a health science that includes these experiences, all we need is a theoretically inclusive basis.

Quantum physics provides us with this much-needed new basis for inclusivity. Quantum physics has given us the long-sought-after science of consciousness, beginning with the idea that consciousness is the ground of all being, of all objects of our experience as well as the self or subject/experiencer. In this ground, quantum objects of experience—sensory material objects, vital energy, and mental meaning—all exist as possibility for consciousness to choose from. This choice is also called downward causation.

We are familiar with experiences manifesting in the brain—both pure thoughts and emotions. In these experiences, consciousness identifies with the brain, an identity we call the ego. Choice actualizes the wave-like many faceted quantum possibility objects into a particle-like single-faceted object of experience. We as the ego-self becomes the observer of the experience. The crucial aspect in this process is the memory-making capacity that the brain has.

What the new data (Item 6, above) is telling us is that there are similar memory-making capacities in the body as well in the heart region and the navel region, which Indians in antiquity named the chakras. This suggests that we can experience pure feelings at these chakras, and that there are self-identities at some of these chakras as well.

Why is this important? When you read the evidence, you will be amazed. Here is a sneak preview. The ordinary experience that many people, especially men, have at the heart, is one of being defensive; the immune system (in the form of the thymus gland function of distinguishing between "me" and "not me") is in charge. However, some people do experience the positive emotion of love there. What gives? The immune system is momentarily suspended for these people, and when that happens, our heart—usually a blood pump—acquires a new function—love.

These aspects of people's experience have been obscure for these reasons: 1) The chakra system has not been taken seriously because there was no theory for it; 2) The thymus gland does most of its defensive work during our early developmental years; once the defense in the form of the lymphatic system is built, it goes somewhat dormant, although not entirely; 3) We have not known about the heart going coherent and quantum until the experimental breakthrough at the Heart Math Institute in California, which has become famous for such groundbreaking research.

This result is most important because it signifies something fantastic: Our physiology is not fixed; our organs can be awakened to pick up additional functions of positivity. Imagine if we could learn to cultivate this trait, how beneficial that would be to our health as a preventive measure. Could cancer be prevented by waking up your heart? Could heart disease? Could Type II diabetes be prevented by awakening the navel chakra and creating a new quantum-stabilized pancreas? Could Alzheimer's be prevented by awakening the brow chakra to be curious, even in old age? A new era of healthcare is about to begin and this book is written in celebration of that, too. We now can include both material and lifestyle effects in our science of health, which we call Quantum Integrative Medicine.

When the Indians and the Chinese codified vital energy, they also realized the importance of this energy to health and healing. Accordingly, they postulated the idea of a vital body and a mental body from which our feelings and thoughts come. When these bodies go awry, they postulated, we get sick, especially the vital body. The healing systems they developed are Ayurveda and Traditional Chinese Medicine, respectively. Today, we put all such medicinal systems under the label of Alternative or Complementary medicine. So you can also think of our book as a scientization of alternative medicine as well as an integration of conventional and alternative medicine.

Conventional medicine is generally evidence-based, but that is not a virtue. The spirit of science—the exploration of Truth—demands that we have both the theory and experimentation to build science. The only theory conventional medicine can claim is germ theory. Alternative medicine systems are based on individual metaphysics and theories that are not entirely scientific. In this book, we propose a genuine science of all medicine with both theoretic and experimental aspects.

I (Amit) attempted earlier to integrate the two systems, but the success of *The Quantum Doctor* was limited by my limited understanding of health issues. Besides, some of the data was not even available yet. Teaming up with Valentina, a medical doctor, and gaining the revelation of new data have helped considerably in improving that earlier effort.

We both promise that this book delivers a viable integrative medicine. It is an outright call for the transformation of healers, patients, and clients—and indeed the entire health-care industry. It is a call for transformation from a disease-oriented mindset to an emphasis on well-being and prevention. A call for an integrative approach to health using a proper science. A call for a change in the attitude that we are born with a fixed system of physiology that cannot be further improved. A call for transformation as well from a mechanistic job-orientation for healers to a transformative orientation. And it is a call for political activism from inside the healing profession against big pharma and the professional organizations that provide it support.

QUANTUM PHYSICS

Objects in quantum physics are objects which exist in two complementary domains:

1. a domain of potentiality in which the quantum objects are waves of possibility;
2. the domain of our familiar space and time, in which quantum objects show their particle nature as their wave potentiality actualizes. In other words, waves consisting of many possibilities (for example, many positions at the same time) change into particle of one actuality (one position at one time).

In Newtonian physics, particles are particles and waves are waves; they are seen as incompatible movements. Particles can only be at one place at a time; even when they move, they describe a trajectory. Waves, on the other hand, spread out and can be in many places at the same time. Both particles and waves are material phenomena in space and time, assumed to be the one and only domain of reality.

Since Newtonian physics came earlier, the prejudice of one domain of reality was already established when quantum physics was discovered. Almost everyone initially thought that the domain of potentiality of quantum physics is metaphysical baggage. Many scientists, a majority maybe, still try to deny its validity.

In 1982, quantum metaphysics, this implicit metaphysical assumption of quantum physics—that there is a domain of potentiality beside the one familiar domain of space and time—became science, not only theory but also verified experimental fact. These experimenters demonstrated faster-than-light communication between quantum objects of potentiality once they interact and correlate, a property called non-locality. Since objects in space and time can only communicate at less than equal to light speed, this experiment is conclusive: the domain of potentiality is outside space and time.

Even earlier, physicist and mathematician John von Newmann had mathematically demonstrated the undeniable observer effect: Only when a human observer (differentiated from inanimate objects by self-awareness) makes a measurement does a quantum wave of potentiality collapse (or actualize) into a particle of actuality. In other words, quantum measurement actualizes the object no doubt, but additionally breaks up the domain of potentiality into a subject (of self-awareness) and an object of experience.

In 1993, in the book *The Self-Aware Universe*, I developed an integrative paradigm of quantum science identifying the domain of potentiality of quantum physics with consciousness as the ground of all being. In this ground, both physical material objects and nonphysical nonmaterial objects can exist as quantum potentialities of consciousness. The physical when manifest gives us the material body; simultaneously, the manifestation of the nonmaterial gives us our nonmaterial bodies. In this way, quantum science provides a metaphysical basis for integration of conventional and alternative medicine.

We have four worlds of experience: physical—sensing, vital—feeling, mental—thinking, and supramental—intuiting. I have not mentioned intuition previously, but it is one of those organ functions for which we need to wake up the chakras. Normally, what you feel at the heart chakra is defensiveness and vulnerability; but when you wake up the heart chakra, the heart awakens to the function of love, which is an intuitive archetype. When you wake up the navel chakra, in addition to the usual security-related feelings of pride and insecurity, feelings of self-worth—an expression of the archetype of love as well—self-love, are experienced. Similarly, if the brow chakra awakens, the neocortex picks up, in addition to rational thinking, the new function of intuitive thinking—an access to the archetypal experiences in general that you did not have before such an awakening.

The ancients thought about this in a simplistic way: There are four worlds of experience giving us a body in each of the worlds, and any of these bodies can get sick. Hence we need a medicine system to help with the healing a sick body. Of course, they left unsolved the not-so-little problem of interaction dualism—how do the different bodies interact with one another? For example, how does a diseased vital body make the physical body sick?

Our experience with computers has given us a monistic metaphor to describe the situation. Computers come as a physical hardware, each component in the hardware follows physical laws. Then, a human operator writes programs with the help of his mind to instruct the various components of the hardware to perform purposive functions. The laws of the program are based on mental logic; they have nothing to do with physical laws.

Physical organs constitute hardware; consciousness creates organ functions as epigenetic programs of instruction to the genes to produce the suitable functional proteins with the help of the potentialities of its vital world. Hence, the software is called vital and the conglomerate of all the vital software is the vital body.

You can think of the cumulation of the memory of each type of experience producing functional software for the physical organ which you must think of as hardware, physiology included, all encased as possibilities in the ground of being of consciousness itself. Human beings have not one but five bodies—this hardware-software combination using the computer analogy (Figure 1). It is just common sense that there could be disease for each of the bodies and that healing for each of these bodies must also be possible. Medicine, to be complete, must deal with all five bodies of the human being.

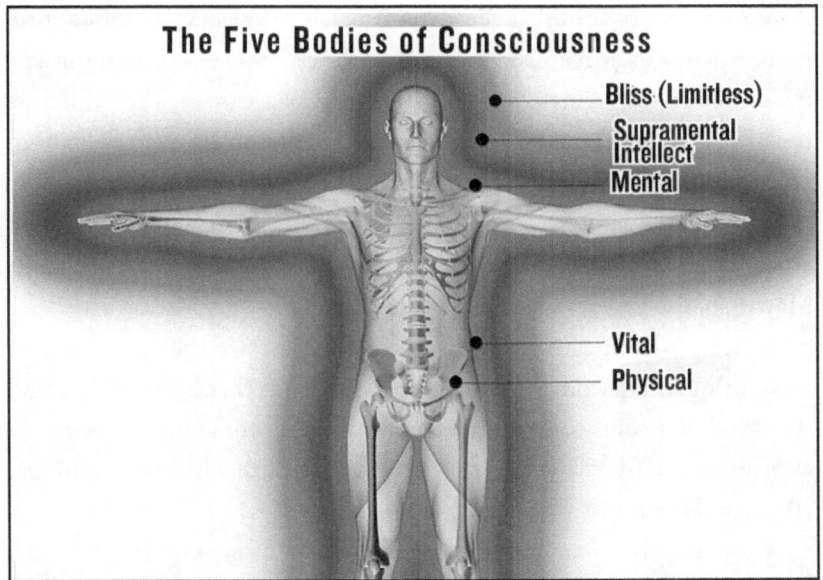

Figure 1. The five bodies of the human being. For good health, each of these bodies needs care.

We all are interested in health and healing and in our physical well-being. We all search for well-being when we don't have it, when we are hit by disease. But with the sharp division of medicine into two camps—conventional and alternative—it is often difficult to choose the proper healing method when we need it. What criteria should we use for such a choice? Is a combination of healing techniques better than any one individual technique? What should we do to maintain our health, to prevent disease in the first place? Can we heal ourselves without any physical or chemical instruments of healing? In the absence of a proper science of medicine, the answers to such questions depend on whom you ask.

Are at least some of those stories of spontaneous healing of cancer and other serious disease true? The experts answer, yes, but is spontaneous healing accessible to all of us? Experts from some medicinal traditions stubbornly shake their heads; others say yes but cannot give convincing guidance as to how.

When we are middle-aged or old, are we destined to suffer from chronic diseases and consider ourselves lucky if we escape without any major debilitating illnesses such as heart disease, cancer, Type II diabetes, or Alzheimer's? Most physicians of either ilk sound optimistic about elder care but cannot back up their optimism with practical techniques of unmitigated success. Should we accept stress, lack of vitality, and chronic disease at old age as the price we must pay for modern living? Maybe so, the experts say. How can this kind of equivocation satisfy?

Experts who suggest remedies propose lifestyles that are too time consuming in relation to health alone. Who has that kind of time and that kind of resolve to heal unless you have a terminal disease? Can we ever discover a lifestyle that gives us optimal health without consuming all our waking hours with health-related activities?

Why is it that we cannot control the play of economics in health matters and the cost of heath goes up and up and up? We are sorry, say experts from both camps. Is medicine only about pathology? Can we not strive for positive health, with vitality and well-being reigning supreme? We don't know, say the experts, with few exceptions.

The truth is, we cannot begin to answer such questions with much credibility without developing an integrative paradigm of the human experience that embraces all medicinal systems that work. We must end the current confusion of paradigms that pervades medicine. Some effort has already begun. After my modest beginning in 2004 with the publication of *The Quantum Doctor*, Dr. Paul Drouin, a conventional medical doctor with impressive alternative medicine credentials, published *Creative Integrative Medicine* in 2014. The physician Larry Dossey has come on board with the idea of the primacy of consciousness; at least partially integrative medicine treatments are now available in several clinics around the world, including the wellness center run by the physician Deepak Chopra. These are all good signs of progress. But these efforts have not gone far enough. Without the benefit of a truly integrative science of medicine and its working, these advancements are not convincing enough.

Quantum integrative medicine, developed here, is based on a truly integrative science of experience; it gives satisfying answers to the questions above, and hopefully will end all paradigm wars in medicine because it is defining a new and consistent paradigm for all of medicine within an integrative overall paradigm of human science.

Is medicine about illness as the majority of the medical establishment still presupposes, or is it about wellness, a new idea that is gradually entering the consciousness of the healing profession and the people they serve? The paradigm of this book settles the issue. Its central theme is that we now have enough knowledge and wisdom to anchor medicine in the concept of wellness and we do this principally by appealing directly to conventional allopathic medicine practitioners and the practitioners of the various forces of alternative medicine to partake in integrative practice and raise people's awareness toward the shift from disease to wellness. We do this by:

- Developing a complete integrative science of health and healing, filling in the gaps of the previous works. In particular, we now have solved the details of how the various nonphysical bodies are manifested. Discovering these details has helped us develop methods of nutrition for all five bodies of the human being, making the idea of preventive medicine a practical one.
- Much of modern medicine's success lies in the development of the concept of external hygiene. This is now being supplemented by the concept of internal hygiene. Internal hygiene not only refers to the internal physical body's environment of the physical cells and organs (blood and other fluids), but also to the vital energy and mental meaning environment, which are generally thought of as our personal unconscious or the subconscious. This is another integration we need to achieve for optimal health, and in this book we show how.
- Helping both healers and their clients shift from a disease mindset to a transformative mindset of well-being. The major shift

required is for the healers to actively engage the archetype of wholeness and integrate their "heads" and their "hearts." Only then can they teach the clients a mindset of exploring wholeness as well through well-being and prevention.
- Solving the problem of chronic disease as one that is for neither conventional or alternative medicine but rather as a problem for everyone to solve. Our solution is twofold. First, if one already has a life-threatening chronic disease, engage creativity and quantum healing.
- For prevention, we are also solving the problem with a new discovery—that human physiology can be changed. And the good news is that we have also discovered how to do this.

Health-profession aspirants, please treat this book as an introduction to an upcoming branch of health profession: quantum health management. Your tool is quantum integrative medicine. Your expertise consists of nutrition for all five bodies for disease prevention, and if disease such as a virus infection happens anyway, you will know how to guide your client into a suitable healing system at the appropriate time; in cases of chronic disease, this would be crucial. Most importantly, you can be a guide and help your client into preventive practices that include changing the harmful physiology built into us as a side effect. You can explore with us the new aborning field of quantum gerontology—preventive care of the elderly in a radically new way.

Consider an almost trivial example of how health management can save a life. In this day of nutritional supplements, patients themselves use supplements without expert advice. In a couple of cases of diabetes, this gave rise to serious problems of allergy via interference with insulin injection. What is the fact? Insulin injection will never heal diabetes. We cannot prevent people from trying alternatives that promise to heal. But by the same token, without some emergency application of insulin, there is too much suffering for the patient. In this way, it is a necessity that there are experts—health managers—who can suggest herbal medicine without interfering with the insulin treatment.

DEFINITIONS

Some definitions are in order, although it is likely that the reader is already familiar with them. Conventional medicine, also called allopathy, is based on the premise that disease is either due to external toxic agents such as germs (bacteria and viruses) or the mechanical malfunctioning of an internal organ of the physical body. In allopathy, a cure is effected mainly by treating the symptoms of the disease until they disappear via drugs, surgery, and, in the case of cancer, energetic radiation. Exotic new techniques, such as gene therapy or nanotechnology, whose premise is to correct the mechanical disorder at the molecular level remain more or less promissory.

In contrast, in mind-body medicine, the premise is that disease is due to a mental problem—for example, mental-emotional stress. The cure is to correct the problem with the mind that will then correct the physiology.

According to the tradition of acupuncture, disease arises because of imbalances in the patterns of vital energy (*chi* in Chinese) flow in the body. The cure consists of correcting these imbalances using puncture at appropriate points of the body with sharp needles. But the energy referred to in acupuncture is nonphysical vital energy, not to be confused with the usual manifestations of physical energy.

Acupuncture is the most famous example of Traditional Chinese Medicine that, in addition to acupuncture, uses special herbs to correct the imbalances of the movements of vital energy.

In homeopathy, the basic idea is "like cures like" in contrast to a cure by an "other" (allopathic drugs developed through trial and error) in allopathy. A substance that produces the same symptoms in a well person as the symptoms of a diseased person is the "like" that cures in homeopathy. But the cure is made downright mysterious by applying the medicinal agent in such dilutions as one part in 10^{30} or even smaller, a process called "dynamization."

Ayurveda is traditional Indian medicine. Thanks to the work of such luminaries as the physician Deepak Chopra, Ayurvedic concepts such as *doshas* have become the subject of parlor games. Who are you, a *vata* person, a *pitta* person, or a *kapha* person? Vata, pitta, and kapha are the Sanskrit names of the three doshas, imbalances of bodily functions and movements that we all have to some degree or other. A unique dominance of one or another dosha, or sometimes a combination of doshas, characterizes each one of us. In fact, we all have a base level amount of each of the doshas. Disease happens when deviations occur taking the body away from our base level of the imbalances, called *prakriti*, at adulthood. Returning the body to the base level of the imbalances, using herbs, massages, cleansing techniques, etc., effects a cure.

Ayurveda is nonmaterial medicine system because the doshas, although physical, are caused by imbalances in how we use nonphysical vital energy as we grow up. Likewise, the herbal remedies work not because of the matter-content but via the efficacy of the vital energy to remedy the vital energy imbalance.

Spiritual healing is the idea of invoking the "higher power" of the Spirit through prayer and other such rituals to heal. Shamanic healing, prayer healing, Christian Science, faith healing, intuitive healing, all fall in this category.

Allopathic physicians have to come to terms with:

- The fact that these alternative healing techniques work;
- What they do, what they heal and how; the imbalances of chi or prana are not about physical substances, but are about a nonphysical substances—vital energy;
- We do have experiences, thinking, feeling, and intuition, which are nonphysical;

- Illness, what people feel when they have a disease, is a nonphysical experience not necessarily identical with the disease;
- The healing of nonphysical experiences cannot be effected by physical causes or interactions, so we must look for nonphysical causes or interactions.

Similarly, alternative medicine practitioners must come to terms with the fact that allopaths will have difficulties in appreciating the value of their trade because they do not use good scientific theories of explanatory power.

- If you are scientifically minded, and you want to understand the relationship of conventional medicine and dosha medicine, you will be disappointed in your readings of the current Ayurvedic literature. In view of the lack of understanding of where doshas originate in conventional medicinal (physiological) terms, the allopath remains skeptical.
- Regarding homeopathy, the conventionalist has to be downright scornful. In the medicinal dilutions that homeopaths prescribe, not even one molecule of the medicine may reach the diseased body. The homeopathic medicine, then, must be regarded as pure "placebo"—an intake of sugar pills disguised as medicine—and the cure then must be considered entirely fortuitous.
- In the same vein, spiritual healing, the idea of relying on Spirit for healing encounters resistance. The Spirit, for an allopath, is a dubious concept, and therefore relying on it is tantamount to relying on the natural processes of the body, which are often inadequate for healing. To do so when all the powerful drugs of allopathy are available seems so preposterous that it drives allopathic practitioners to utter frustration. Of course, allopaths too often forget the severe side effects that pharmaceutical medicines often produce.

Let's also remember that the practitioners of alternative medicine are equally scornful of allopathic practices. Allopathic drugs are mostly poisons to the body with harmful side effects. Why should we poison the body when alternatives are available? For chronic and degenerative diseases especially, allopathy is ineffective anyway. It merely cures the symptoms but does not heal the real cause which is nonphysical. Finally, allopathic medicine is not cost effective. As the reader surely knows, it is largely the economics of allopathic medicine that is making people look for alternatives in medicine.

How do we go from these deep divisions among the practitioners of the two camps to an integral medicine that both camps can accept? The answer is that we have to go to the philosophical roots of all the medicine practices and discover their unifying bridge-building philosophy. That work began in *The Quantum Doctor*. Here, we present the current depths of unification available to medicine practitioners of both camps from the point of view of prevention.

A NEW BIOLOGY OF CONSCIOUSNESS, FEELING, MEANING, AND PURPOSE

Traditional biology misses it all. Neither feeling nor meaning let alone purpose can be included in materialist molecular biology even when supplemented by Neo-Darwinism which, unfortunately, is also neither here nor there.

Molecular biology or the more recent biology of cellular automata looks at life as information processing of living programs—machine living. Supplement this with programs of artificial intelligence machines. You've got a machine doing programmed living and thinking. What is lacking? The living and thinking experience. There is no self or subject in the programs that experiences anything.

There is always that question of subject/self that will perpetually haunt the researcher of artificial life or intelligence or a combo.

What about Neo-Darwinism and all the philosophical claims that come with it? The contention of bio-philosophers seems to be that given the four billion years of Darwinian evolution and the organisms' struggles for survival; anything can happen to the organism that has survival advantage. The list includes feeling, meaning, even consciousness. Of course, nobody ever demonstrates anything (except the biologists who work with cellular automata, or at least they try). Instead, these bio-philosophers' work well illustrates what the philosopher Karl Popper called "promissory materialism."

The truth about Neo-Darwinism is this: There seems to be no way to give a materialist molecular basis to the Darwinian idea that nature selects among gene mutations on the basis of what will help survivability of the species. In the 1970s there was some research by the biologist Manfred Eigen and others to produce in the laboratory "molecules of living"—DNA, RNA, and protein—that thrive to survive starting from the nonliving. The initial research was promising; but nobody ever succeeded all the way. No one has produced a single molecule in the laboratory with survivability built into it starting from the nonliving alone. Nonliving molecules and their conglomerates do not try to survive, which is a property of the living.

Neo-Darwinism projects a tantalizing amount of explanatory power when used with appropriate sophistry. However, it does not uphold scientific materialism; it cannot connect to molecular biology as argued in the previous paragraph.

And of course, every critic of Neo-Darwinism knows that this theory cannot explain experimental data either: The gaps in the continuity of fossil data and species evolving from simple to complex are only the most glaring. (Read Amit's book *Creative Evolution* for details.)

Work on new biology has already begun. The biologist Bruce Lipton has written an evocative book, *The Biology of Belief*. This book contributes toward a new understanding of what life is. And Amit's book *Creative Evolution* develops an evolutionary biology based on the primacy of consciousness integrating ideas of quantum physics with ideas of two spiritual bio-philosophers, Sri Aurobindo and Teilhard de Chardin.

On the theoretical side, what Neo-Darwinism lacks is the recognition that evolution of the genes and development of the organs of purposive functions from the genes—require separate mechanisms. Biologists are gradually recognizing that evolution is really Evo-Devo—evolution and development together. This, too, has been accomplished in the quantum theory giving us a theory of emotions in the brain as well as in the body, including the experience of feelings in body centers of the chakras. In this way, quantum biology gives us an adequate scientific basis for an integrative quantum science of health and healing.

A new healing manifesto for the client: Be your own quantum doctor most of the time with occasional help from an integrative health management practitioner.

Quantum integrative medicine has two aspects: It is an integrative medicine for the healer to use and a preventive medicine for the client to practice with only occasional guidance from the healer.

Here is more good news for the client. The quantum worldview empowers you, and says that the power to heal, which physicians call the placebo, is your power. Disease means, in part, that somehow the stress of everyday living has confused you to give up your power. The idea that your doctor, and the medicine she prescribes, will heal restores your power. This is how placebos work.

What does this power actually consist of? It is the ability to align your intentions with the healing power that your vital physical body already has, that it already uses regularly to keep you healthy within certain limits, provided that you don't give up on your healing intention. In truth, your healing power goes way beyond this. In truth, you can literally choose health over disease if you develop the necessary skillful means of living that we introduce in this book.

Meanwhile, let us share with you a touching anecdote of a brave woman. The physician Andrew Weil has cited the case of the patient designated as "S.R.," who was diagnosed with Hodgkin's disease (a cancer of the lymphatic system) in his book *Health and Healing*. Hodgkin's disease is known to progress in four stages. S.R. was already in stage three. She was pregnant at the time and did not want to lose the baby, so she refused conventional treatment with radiation or chemotherapy and found a new doctor. Under his supervision, she had surgery, even radiation treatment, but the situation continued to worsen.

It just so happened that this woman's physician was researching the application of LSD therapy for cancer patients. Under his guidance, she took a guided LSD trip during which the doctor encouraged her to go deep inside herself and communicate with the life in her womb. It was then that S.R. had a sudden flash of insight and realized that she had the choice to live or die. It took a while after this illumination, a lot of lifestyle changes to be sure, but she was healed. Incidentally, she also gave birth to a healthy child.

According to the quantum worldview, every one of us has this choice only if we learn to exercise it via a purposive life full of the Seven Is: Inspiration, Intention, Intuition, Imagination, Incubation, Insight, and Implementation. It is through our experiences of intuition and insight that we know that we have become aligned with the purposive movement of consciousness.

REDEFINING THE ROLE OF THE DOCTOR OR HEALER

For arriving at a redefinition of the role of the patient that preventive medicine demands, it is imperative that we redefine the more recent concept of the objective (machine-like) physician that we currently have.

I (Amit) always chuckle when I remember an incident that an allopathic doctor reported at a medical conference at the University of Oregon. When the doctor asked his patient, "How are you feeling?" his patient retorted, "That's for you to tell me." A robotic answer on the part of the patient, no doubt. But the joke is on whom because there is a rationale for the patient's response? The patient knows that there were a bunch of tests done on his blood and whatever else and the doctor will treat him accordingly following the prevalent machine wisdom.

If material monism is right, and both the doctor and the patient are machines, then all this discussion is irrelevant and robots are going to replace machines anyway in the near future. We know from direct experience and from the results of Alain Aspect's experiment (in quantum mechanics) that we are conscious beings who have a choice, so why go on pretending that we are machines? Truly, some patients would love to have the doctor take the entire responsibility for their health. But can doctors handle it? And should they?

At an advanced stage of my spiritual practice, a teacher told me to take responsibility for the "other." This is what a healer has to do when he interacts with patients. This is standard empathy practice and, indeed, all healers would be better healers if they developed it. Yet in Western culture, the average physician is almost as far from empathic relationships as the patients are.

Should we include empathy training—the quantum way—in a medical doctor's training? You bet. With new understanding of our "feeling" selves—traditionally called the "heart"—it is not even hard. It is what some people call having an open heart. And even so, wouldn't it be much better if patients handled and shared some of the burden of maintaining their health too? Preventive medicine does that also.

DEVELOPING A GENERAL THEORY OF HEALTH AND WELL-BEING

The practice of medicine has never been fully scientific. This is true for modern allopathic medicine as well. Science requires two complementary aspects: theory and experiment. Theory alone is mere philosophy; inspired though it may be, it has to undergo experimental verification in order to be reliable; empirical data alone cannot give us the full context in which to evaluate the data. In other words, the evidence-based medicine that masquerades as medical science today is faulty, half-truth.

We all sympathize with the desperation that calls for evidence-based medicine in both allopathic and alternative medicine. Except for germ theory, and for disease, there is no real theory in conventional medicine.

Even for a simple thing like a cut finger, we cannot answer the question why simply applying a bandage not only stops the bleeding but also mends the skin to its previous condition through regeneration. In allopathy and conventional biology, it is impossible to define the concept of integrity of human body parts or organs or explain regeneration.

But that is one of the outstanding achievements of Quantum Integrative Medicine. Using quantum biology, not only can we define the integrity of body organs and define optimal health as the harmonious dynamic functioning of all of the five bodies that we are born with, but we can also change our physiology for the better and build a new body—and soul—to show for it.

How far can we take this line of thinking? Quite far, as you will see. In this book, our aim is no less than to develop a general theory of human health and well-being.

Science is theory and experiment working hand-in-hand. How far have we come in the science of diagnosis of disharmony between the different bodies? Quite far. Even so, healing science will continue to need complementary help from healing arts.

PART ONE

A NEW PERSPECTIVE for the SCIENCE of MEDICINE

chapter one

HARDWARE AND SOFTWARE: WHY WE NEED TO INCLUDE MORE THAN THE MATERIAL BODY FOR HEALTHCARE AND QUANTUM INTEGRATIVE MEDICINE TO WORK

Traditional Eastern medicine is still practiced in China and India, and other Asian countries. Let's consider this mainstay in much of alternative medicine to understand modern medicine's most glaring omission.

Eastern cultures, in their traditional healing practices, use such concepts as the flow of chi in Chinese medicine (*ki* in Japanese) or *prana* in Indian Ayurveda. In ancient treatises it is quite clear what chi or prana is—some sort of energy, but nonmaterial. Yet in modern expositions of these subjects, especially in the West, our experience is that nobody is very clear on what chi or prana means. For instance, it is left vague whether chi or prana is a physical or a nonphysical entity. Most modern authors pussyfoot around the meaning of these concepts because they cannot explain them in terms that are acceptable to modern materialist science's worldview.

There is actually a corresponding concept called "vital energy" in the West, but it conjures up the image of a dualistic philosophy of vitalism, a philosophy that biologists discarded some time ago in favor of molecular biology. In general, researchers and scientists in the West, and even healers using alternative medicine, are reluctant (afraid?) to use the phrase "vital energy." Instead, they opt to use the phrase "subtle energy" and most of them persist in their materialist beliefs about what subtle energy is—the energy of movements subtler than we have discovered so far but material. Some look at subtle energy as holistic—an emergent phenomenon of the living cells and organs of the body.

Many people think of subtle energy as energy of a higher frequency than gross physical energy. In his book *Vibrational Medicine*, Dr. Richard Gerber says that the difference between physical and subtle matter lies in a simple frequency difference. This is confusing, and wrong, in fact, because it tempts you to think that physical and subtle matter are made of the same basic substance. But this is categorically wrong because matter is reducible to smaller bits, whereas the subtle is not.

One has to go no further than to consider homeopathy to convince oneself that there have to be nonphysical agents at play in at least some cases of healing. In homeopathy, a medicinal substance is applied (orally) in such a diluted proportion that scientific calculations show without a doubt that not one molecule of the "medicine" may find its way to the treatment center of the disease. And yet, the success of homeopathy seems to hold up, even in double-blind clinical trials, which are also designed in such a way as to make sure that homeopathy is not a mere placebo. So, if the efficacy of homeopathy is true, then there must be agents of healing that are nonphysical. We have to come to terms with the idea of nonphysical agents of healing.

In this way, I (Amit) realized very soon after I started research that alternative healing practices remain a mystery (and, therefore, controversial) to most people of conventional thinking because their proponents suffer from five metaphysical shortcomings:

1. There is a lack of distinction between mind and consciousness.
    a. Long ago, Descartes put the two concepts, mind and consciousness, together as the one concept of mind, and that error still haunts medicine.
    b. The causal role of consciousness as the origin of down-

ward causation is either missed or obscured in ambiguity. Somehow, the lessons of quantum physics have not penetrated the Newtonian physics armor of practitioners of alternative medicine.
2. The distinctive role of the mind as opposed to the brain is missed.

    Philosophical progress in this field—the idea that the material brain cannot process mental meaning (read John Searle's book *The Rediscovery of the Mind*), which is already decades old—has been missed. And therefore scientific progress—that fMRI measurements can reveal the workings of the mental software of the brain hardware—has been missed.
3. The vital body's distinctive role in providing the epigenetic nonlocal component of organ physiology has also been missed. Recent scientific progress about bioelectric body and measurability of vital energy has been missed also.
4. Neither consciousness, nor the mind, nor the vital body, even if acknowledged, whether they are nonphysical is left ambiguous.
5. The role of creativity, that the body and the brain's physiology can be drastically improved, has not yet entered the medical mindset—not even for practitioners of alternative medicine.

We also have to solve the problem of dualism, but who says that there is no way to get around dualism, that it is an insurmountable problem? On the other hand, it is just common sense that during the development of the embryo, nonlocal instant coordination between different organs is essential. Material objects can never simulate nonlocality.

It is through solving these knotty problems of philosophy that I (Amit) arrived at a science within consciousness for medicine, Quantum Integrative Medicine, which I initiated in my book *The Quantum Doctor* and which Valentina and I are bringing to the next level of completion in this book. The experimental techniques and their findings have been a welcome surprise.

Our integrative paradigm acknowledges and includes the rediscovery of downward causation by consciousness in quantum physics. It also takes advantage of the rediscovery of the mind and the vital body within science. It then uses quantum thinking as a way of introducing the mental and vital bodies in medicine as distinct from the physical and without falling prey to dualism. Finally, the mental and the vital in quantum science bring us infinite potentiality to heal as well as build new improved software via quantum creativity. This is our crowning achievement.

INTEGRATION

Material healing is healing through upward causation, and spiritual and subtle healing is healing through downward causation, but how do we incorporate the details of mind-body healing or subtle or vital energy healing in our integrative paradigm?

When consciousness collapses a material wave of possibility, we manifest the experience of sensing as part of our material body experience. So how does our experience of thinking arise? Ordinary thinking must be the result of collapsing a possibility wave of the mind—our mental body. Similarly, collapsing a "possibility wave" of vital energy, a movement of the vital body, gives us the experience of feeling. And intuition is the way we experience still another category of possibilities of consciousness: its revealing aspects, which we will refer to generically as the archetypes of the supramental domain.

But materialists object. We know that thinking most often involves memories which are stored in the brain. There is no experience of the mind without the brain. So how do we know that thinking is not a brain phenomenon?

Looking at the mind and the brain as a software-hardware combo solves the problem. Consciousness uses the mental possibilities of meaning to make mental software that the brain assigns symbols like a computer.

In the same vein, how do we know that the possibilities whose collapse gives us the experience of feeling, does not belong to the physical body itself? Aren't emotions associated with the response to special stimuli of the nervous system in the midbrain? Do we really need to postulate the vital body? Yes, we do. It is true that the brain takes over and controls the body organ's normal software. Hence, the emotions we normally experience are from the brain circuits in the midbrain causing confusion.

WHAT DOES THE VITAL BODY DO THAT THE PHYSICAL CANNOT DO?

The rediscovery of the vital body took place in the 1980s when a crucial step occurred in the work of the biologist Rupert Sheldrake. In 1981 he proposed an explanation of the hitherto unexplained phenomenon of morphogenesis—biological form- and organ-making in terms of nonphysical and nonlocal morphogenetic fields residing outside space and time. His work was originally intended to explain the phenomenon of cell differentiation—how living cells belonging to different organs but containing the same DNA manage to make different proteins for their purposive functions—but he also clarified the role of the vital body that now can be seen to be the abode of the morphogenetic fields as distinct from the physical: It is to provide the software programs for the organ hardware. Consciousness uses the morphogenetic fields as blueprints to make epigenetic vital software.

What no physical interactions can do are form the purposive physiological functions that the biological forms—the organs—perform. Purpose lies outside the jurisdiction of materialist science, and here is where we need to invoke nonphysical organizing fields as the source of vital software for programming biological organs for performing purposive biological functions. Since the vital software is designed to enable organ functions, such as maintenance of the body, reproduction, etc., let's call the morphogenetic fields by the applied name for this context, "morphogenetic/liturgical fields" (*liturgical* is the Greek word for functional), or simply, the liturgical fields.

When consciousness simultaneously collapses the possibility waves of the physical organ and its vital correlate (Figure 2), what we experience is the feeling of the vital energy of movement of the morphogenetic/liturgical blueprints of an organ's vital software.

Many authors have noted that all the important organs of the body are situated along the spine and its imaginary continuation through the brain (Figure 3), and the previously mentioned chakras are found close to important organs of the physical body. Now we see why. The chakras are the places where we experience the feelings associated with the collapse of the physical-vital hardware-software of the most important organs of our body. This vital software, correlated with the physical organs, is universal, common to all humans.

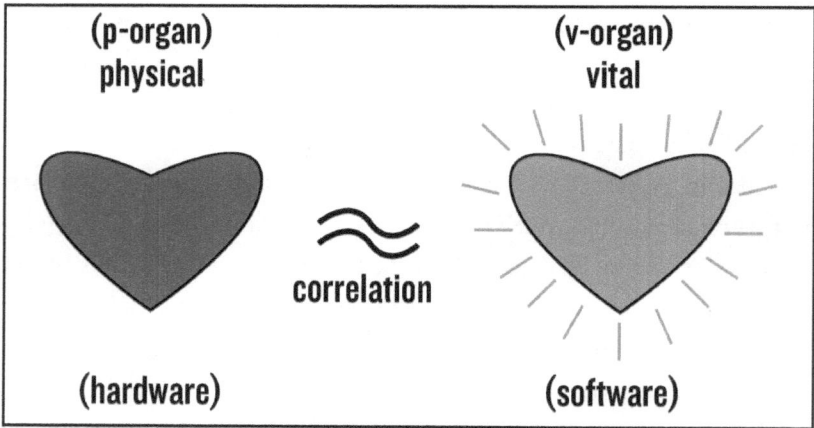

Figure 2. Every physical organ and its physiology has a correlated vital software (V-organ) to program the physiology into the organ hardware.

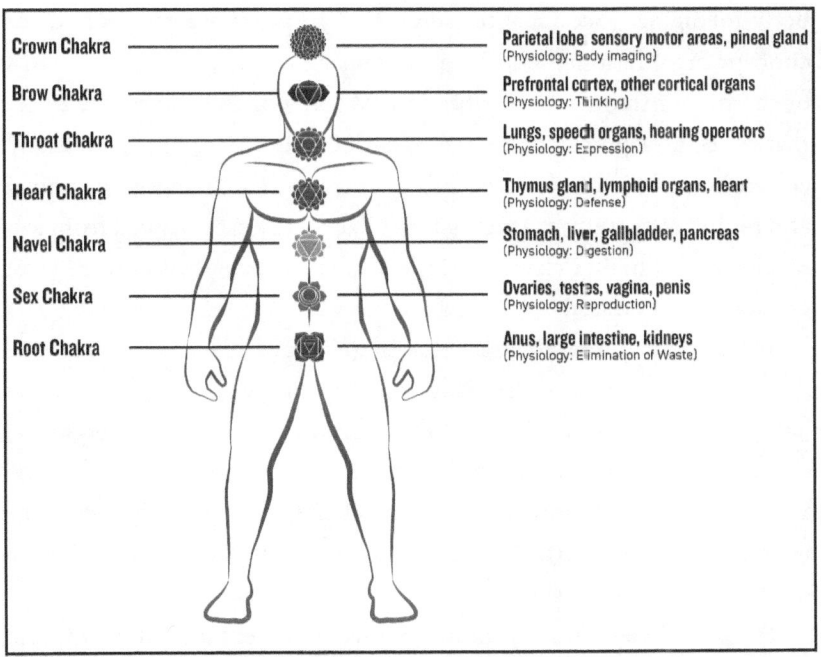

Figure 3. All the important organs of the body are located along the spine and its imaginary extension through the brain. Each group has an associated chakra.

Of course, once we have the universal vital software in the midbrain, it is easy to forget their origin—the morphogenetic/liturgical fields and the vital software of the body organs. Here, you have to remember creativity, creative healing of a disease—organ malfunction. In creative healing, we actualize new liturgical fields to program new vital software from previously unactualized liturgical fields to restore the organ function.

As an example, consider cancer, which is an immune system malfunction brought about by the immune system's inability to kill off cancerous cells. In spontaneous healing without medical intervention, patients spontaneously take a creative quantum leap to make new vital software that restores the immune system with such great causal efficacy that a malignant tumor disappears overnight.

The rediscovery of vitality leads to the concept of vital creativity. Indeed, the chakras and vital creativity play important roles in vital body medicine. (See Chapters 8 and 17.) Earlier, we mentioned the concept of vibrational medicine—seeing subtle energy as gross energy of the higher frequency of vibration. We now invite the reader to see that work as a precursor to the scientific concept of chakras as conceived here. Instead of seeing subtle energy as gross energy of higher and higher frequency, try seeing it as vital energy experienced from low to higher and higher chakras—indeed, there is progression from gross to subtler and subtler.

In the first three chakras, the energies are reflective of survival issues—maintenance of the body and reproduction. At the heart, it is love, which is much subtler. At the throat and the brow, the energies are expressing abstract archetypes like truth and justice, very subtle. And at the crown, when properly understood, the energies truly reflect the feelings associated with the subtle bodies alone, when detached from the gross physical altogether.

For good health, it is essential to experience feelings in the body and know your chakras, however foreign the concepts of vital energy and chakras may seem. In the 1980s when ideas like vital energy and chakras had just begun to percolate into the Western psyche, I (Amit) remember getting a call from the University of Oregon Psychology Department asking me to help evaluate a man who was claiming to demonstrate vital energy to them. I went there to find a man who seemed pleasant albeit a little frustrated. He was repeatedly rubbing his palms together and asking the people present (mostly skeptical behavioral psychologists) to put their hands in the space between his palms without touching them. Then he would ask, "Are you feeling anything?" to which, one by one, all the psychologists said, "No." But when I put my hand in the space between his palms, I immediately felt strong tingles. When I shared that with my psychologist colleagues, they still would not believe. They thought I was being naive.

HARDWARE AND SOFTWARE

THE REDISCOVERY OF THE MIND

Can computers think? Today suitably programmed computers can carry on a conversation with us thinking humans, so how can we deny computers' capacity for thinking? And, since the brain seems to be a thinking computer, why should we doubt that thinking originates in the brain itself?

Materialists contend that nonphysical mind is not needed as a separate concept. Not so fast, cautioned the philosopher John Searle, who, in the 1980s, argued against a thinking computer. Searle's argument was basically that computers are symbol-processing machines. They cannot process meaning. Thinking involves not only the processing of information that can be codified as symbols but also the processing of meaning. So, computers do not think.

But if we reserve some of the symbols for processing meaning, we need to reserve more symbols to process the meaning of the meaning symbols, and then ever more symbols for processing the meaning of the meaning of the meaning symbols, ad infinitum. So there never are enough symbols for the computer to succeed to process meaning starting from scratch. How do we humans do it, then? We use our minds.

The mathematician Roger Penrose gave a rigorous proof of Searle's idea using Gödel's incompleteness theorem: An elaborate system of mathematical logic is either inconsistent or incomplete. So the mind being needed as a separate nonmaterial entity that processes meaning is the only way we can make sense of what is. Thinking requires a separate mental body. We have it, and this is why we can think.

If material movements are possibilities, then it makes sense to posit that mental movements are meaning possibilities. When we choose from the meaning possibilities, we have a concrete thought of unique meaning which can be represented as a symbol: information. Consciousness, in every experience, not only has a physical perception of a physical object, but also a mental cognition of the meaning of the object. Matter and mind are both possibilities of consciousness. When consciousness converts these possibilities in a collapse event of actual experience, some of the possibilities are collapsed as physical and some as mental. In this way, nonlocal consciousness clearly is seen as the mediator of the interaction between mind and body, and there is no dualism. And now room is made for mind-body healing in which a proper role is given to consciousness (the causal agent of downward causation), and to mind (from which meaning comes), in relation to the physical body and its healing. Think of the brain as computer hardware that consciousness uses via mental software.

From a quantum point of view, it is not hard to see why the mind and meaning are important in medicine. Ordinarily we live in an individual separate reality, distinct from the wholeness of consciousness. It is our mental conditioning that gives us individuality. There is no one-to-one correspondence between objects and their meaning. It is only our mental conditioning that makes it appear so. No wonder we are fooled to believe in independent separate objects. From this separatist point of view, we can partake in actions that can increase our sense of separateness and contract consciousness (as when we assign limited conditioned meaning to our experience) or we can engage in actions that expand consciousness (as when we creatively discover new meaning). The former is subtle suffering, of course, but we may not immediately see it. Contracted consciousness becomes a comfortable cocoon because of familiarity. Disease is a reminder—like being hit by a two-by-four, to be sure—to change our ways, to reverse the journey toward wholeness where healing takes us.

Giving incorrect subjective meaning to objective facts of physical reality is responsible for today's political polarization; however, that makes little difference to our health. But when we give wrong meaning to an experience of feeling producing a wrong emotion uncalled for, it is a different story altogether, for this produces emotional stress, and emotional stress has been linked with much of chronic disease.

THE SUPRAMENTAL BODY: SOUL-MAKING

When we investigate the creativity of the mind, we find that creativity at the low level consists of finding new meaning, a shift of mental meaning from conditioned old ones to an innovative new one—invention—but without changing the archetypal context. This is called situational creativity. But at the highest level, creativity consists of discontinuous leaps in the archetypal context of thinking as well. This is called fundamental creativity and it consists of discovery; here, we are discovering the fundamental laws of movement of the different worlds already present in the compartment of consciousness called supramental, which we have forgotten and can access only through intuitions and creative insights. In contrast, situational creativity is invention and accessible, at least in principle, to reason. Invention depends on the discoveries of fundamental creativity, but not vice versa.

The existence of fundamental creativity points us to the existence of the supramental world. Note, however, that the supramental world is not only the reservoir of the contexts of mental meaning but also of vital functions and physical laws.

We humans have not evolved the capacity of making direct representation of the supramental archetypes onto the physical. We manage with the thoughts and feelings that an archetype evokes, making mental and vital representations (memories) of the archetypes in the process. The totality of these representations can be thought of as our supramental body. Some traditions call it a soul; others call it a higher mind, but, of course, a higher vital must also be involved. In this way, the soul consists of the software of higher mind as well as positive emotional circuits in the body and the brain.

We are not born with much of a soul; the normal biological body does not come with it. You have to make it. Is it worth it? In this book, we show that a few basic aspects of soul-making are already available to us, in our collective unconscious, that we culturally ignore and suppress. We can learn not to do that and instead creatively explore it. We also present the rudiments of the science and art of soul-making that is the key to growing old with quality of life intact.

Caution: the word "soul" also denotes the supposed surviving entity after our death in many religions. We are using the word here to denote soul as part of the great chain of being (physical) body, vital body, mind, soul (supramental body), and Spirit (quantum self).

THE BLISS BODY

When we meditate, we relax—the relaxation response—and we are blissful. But there is new evidence of bliss outside of meditation. Under the guidance of the transpersonal psychiatrist Stan Grof, many people have discovered blissful states akin to *samadhi* through the use of psychedelic drugs and holotropic breathing. Others have discovered blissful states in near-death experiences. These experiences are validating the ancient (Indian) description of consciousness as an existence-awareness-bliss trio. Of this trio, existence is the most immediately obvious element; most of us do not deny awareness (even neuroscientists now think that in the least, we are philosophical robots—in other words, robots with experiences), but high levels of bliss used to be somewhat removed from the everyday experience of people. Not anymore, and this is helping change the worldview.

We momentarily live in the bliss body whenever we leap to the quantum self, a deeper state of our self-experience that arises when we are in the present moment. Neuroscientists have discovered that the brain goes into a nonlocal mode of functioning whenever this happens; many brain areas act in synchrony, as if functioning together as one led by a conductor of an orchestra, the conductor being the quantum self whose baton is nonlocality. And indeed, long-term meditators who make frequent forays to the quantum self can develop this quantum mode of functioning as if it is a trait as can be seen in the book *Altered Traits* by Daniel Goleman and Richard Davidson. So these long-term meditators can be said to have a well-developed bliss body.

HARDWARE AND SOFTWARE

INTEGRATING WESTERN AND EASTERN WAYS OF HEALING

The new idea of organs as a vital-physical correlated body demonstrates the promise of integrating Western and Eastern medicine. Yes, the physical body chemistry is important, as is the hardware of the computer, so conventional medicine is important. But also important are the correlated vital body movements that consciousness actualizes, along with the physical body organs and their physiology—programmed functions.

In general, wellness requires the dynamic homeostasis of physical hardware and vital software; our feelings at the chakras can tell us if the organs at the chakra are functioning properly or not. Why dynamic? Because of environmental factors—both physical and emotional—the organ functions are always changing within a certain range. In any given situation, consciousness needs to actualize the appropriate software program; it must be free to choose accordingly. If the appropriate choice is blocked, we feel disharmony.

Eastern medicine concentrates more on the lack of balance and harmony of the vital body movements that we experience as feelings. In Traditional Chinese Medicine this is an imbalance of the yin and yang aspects of vital energy chi, the wave and particle aspects of chi respectively, if you will. This is vague, to be sure, but it gives us a big hint.

We operate in two different modes of self-identity: the ego or the Newtonian mode and the quantum self or the quantum mode. In the Newtonian mode, we are localized and determined; we can call it the particle mode of identity. In the quantum mode, we are nonlocal and free; we can recognize it as the wave mode. So, balancing the modes of movement of the vital body means balancing the conditioned Newtonian and the creative quantum modes of self-identity in the operations of vital body movements.

In other words, according to Traditional Chinese Medicine, a balance of actuality (yang) and creative potentiality (yin) of chi is needed for the proper maintenance of health. The actual function needed from an organ changes due to environment, change of seasons, bacterial or viral infection, emotional stress, etc. The organ software can be adjusted to the need via situational creativity depending upon the available yin. In other words, if there is adequate yin, consciousness makes permutations and combination of the available potentiality to make a new software that fits the situation Too little yin will reduce the capacity for creative situational adjustment of the software. On the other hand, too little conditioned yang will also decrease creativity because the creative ability is not being engaged. This is why a dynamic creative yin-conditioned yang balance is the recipe for vital wellness.

A dynamic homeostasis is to be maintained where situational creative forays outside the same conditioned response of the vital body are taking place as needed.

The Eastern traditions of medicine see illnesses (especially chronic ones) as due to the imbalance in the way vital body movements occur. All Eastern traditions believe in reincarnation. In their schema, people can be born with certain traits in the manner vital movements are regularly employed. If vital body movements are employed in an unbalanced way to begin with (think of this as vital body karma), with more yin or more yang, they will produce faulty functioning in the physical organs sooner or later. If further vital body imbalance is produced in this life, then there will be further lack of synchrony between the correlated vital and physical states and the functions they perform.

When you have a physical ailment like a headache, the Western physician looks for analgesics that will relieve the symptom, the pain. The Eastern acupuncturist, on the other hand, will try to find a way of correcting the particular imbalance between the yin and yang functioning of the vital body that is the root cause of the pain. So the acupuncturist empirically discovers the particular point of the physical body to probe with the acupuncture needle that will throw a monkey wrench in the faulty conditioned movements of the vital body. The acupuncture probe is designed to be a trigger that will initiate the correctional mechanism for the vital imbalance.

If you are suffering from fatigue, from a lack of vitality, Western medical practitioners will look for a cause, such as anemia or hypoglycemia, and once again, treat the symptoms once they are clearly diagnosed. But if you go to a doctor trained in the Indian Ayurvedic tradition, this doctor will treat you with herbal medicines that are designed to correct your pranic imbalance. Through empirical research and experience, the Ayurvedic physician knows the herb or combination of herbs most likely to help restore the balance of the pranic movements needed for the healing of your particular ailment.

Built into the Eastern philosophy of healing is this: There are special people, spiritual healers, who can institute vital body healing by merely touching or making a sweeping gesture with their hands over the body of the patient. Fortunately, such "hands-on healing" is not restricted to Eastern medicine alone; many spiritual traditions in the West use it, and people with special healing powers are revered in these traditions.

SUMMARY

In brief, considerations of quantum physics tell us the following about the nature of our whole being:

- Consciousness is the ground of all being.
- Matter, vital energies, mental meaning, and supramental archetypes are all quantum possibilities of consciousness. Consciousness mediates the interaction between these worlds of possibility within itself and there is no dualism.

Note: How does consciousness mediate the interaction between two of our bodies, for example, the physical and the vital? By collapsing their chosen actuality (from possibility) simultaneously (Figure 4).

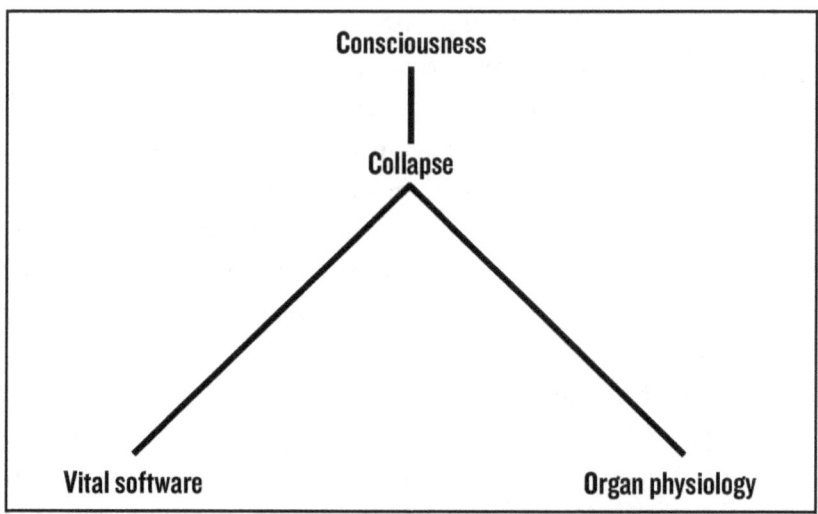

Figure 4. Consciousness mediates between vital and physical bodies by collapsing their possibility waves simultaneously.

- We have not one but five different bodies (see Figure 1): 1) the physical body (hardware plus physiology), sometimes called the gross body (because it looks so stable and permanent in the macro level); 2) the lower vital body—the conglomeration of all the vital software either in conjunction of physical-vital or in the form of physical-vital-mental (negative emotion and pleasure); 3) the lower mental body or simply the mind consisting of the mental software correlated with the brain physical memory; and 4) the supramental body, consisting of physical hardware/ higher vital/higher mental (positive emotional) software (also called the soul), and, together, all these types of subtle software are sometimes called the subtle body (because their dynamic is constantly changing); and 5) the ground of being experienced as the bliss of forever new quantum self, sometimes called the causal body (because it is the doorway to the causal source of downward causation).

DISEASE AND ILLNESS

It is useful to distinguish between disease and illness. Disease is objective malfunctioning of the organism that can be diagnosed by machines, by suitable tests about which one can form a consensus. In contrast, illness is subjective, it is the subjective feeling of the malfunctioning. The materialist paradigm tries to explain disease but lacks the scope to explain the cause of the inner feeling or illness.

So, disease is external, it is telling us about the physical body—hardware and physiology. Illness is internal—it is telling us about the malfunctioning of the simultaneously experienced correlated psyche. If there were a one-to-one correspondence between disease and illness, there would be no problem; treating the disease would automatically treat the illness and vice versa. But empirically, there is no one-to-one correspondence: we can have a disease (early stages of cancer) but not feel ill. Or we can feel ill (having so-called psychosomatic pain), but there is no physical disease that we can find to be its cause. This is why we need an integrative medicine whose aim is not only to cure a disease as well as to heal the feeling of illness.

Quantum integrative medicine gives you the medical science (theory and evidence-based) of maintaining health of all five of our bodies, and in case of both disease and illness, old and new methods of healing.

THE LEVELS OF DISEASE AND HEALING

The physical level of disease seems easy to talk about: it is the body's normal physics and chemistry gone awry. The causes can be both external and internal. Examples of external cause are things like germs, viruses, and physical injuries.

The internal causes of a physical disease are more subtle, but one obvious one is a genetic defect—the deficiency of a gene or a combination of genes translates into the body's incapacity to make particular proteins for proper organ functioning—hence the disease.

But such an analysis for the cause of a disease is not always possible. Take the case of cancer, for example. Both germ theory and gene deficiency have been tried as cause, but without much success. So the question of what causes cancer is quite open to theories at the vital and the mental levels.

What causes disease at the vital level? At the physical level, we have the physical body hardware and physiology, subject to usual physics and chemistry; at the vital level we have the vital software—functional programs that run the physiology according to the repeated use of blueprints of the liturgical fields. Some of the software is universal, but there is also a personal component due to the body's development from childhood to adulthood. Each individual physical body is unique because of its structure. An individual's vital body is also unique but for a different reason: the individual nature of development. Certain vital blueprints and programs are used more than others; many propensities become the pattern of a functional personality. Such an individual vital body 1) may have certain imbalances built into it (internal cause) or may acquire imbalances due to interactions with the physical, the vital, and the mental environments (external cause) or 2) may acquire dynamic imbalance between creativity and conditioning.

Such an environment may consist of food, nature, animals, and other people. Note that interactions with the physical and mental environment are both indirect and direct. Physical environment affects the physical body organs. But the latter are correlated with the vital body software which must adjust, and so the effect propagates. Of course, consciousness makes the ultimate connection. Similarly, the mental environment affects the correlated brain apparatuses and their V-organs. The brain is connected to the various organs of the physical body through the nervous system and also through newly discovered psycho-neuro-immunological and psycho-neuro-gastrointestinal molecular connections. Finally, these organs are correlated with the vital body blueprints at the appropriate chakras. And consciousness can always make direct connection nonlocally.

These imbalances of the vital software (the liturgical fields conditioned through repeated use) and their movements (associated with the running of the functional programs) then produce imbalances in the physical organ function as well that can produce even structural problems (such as the growth of a tumor).

At the mental level, negative meaning may be attributed to external input occurring at all three levels:

1. At the physical level. For example, an injury causing mental anguish: "Why do bad things always happen to me?"
2. At the vital feeling level. For example, the sight of a difficult boss producing mental fantasy fears as potent as the fear arising from seeing a real tiger.
3. At the mental-emotional level. For example, hearing words of insult.

Negative mental meaning affects the vital body software in the brain directly through the brow chakra—which covers the neocortex—and through a lesser-known chakra at the midbrain and the correlated organs of hypothalamus and the pituitary gland, and vital software at the body chakras indirectly through the psycho-neuro-immunological and psycho-neuro-gastrointestinal connections.

Additionally, the mind of an individual may also have built-in internal imbalances. Both internal and external imbalances of the mind are able to produce vital as well as physical imbalances.

Since the archetypal supramental level is not directly represented in the physical, there are not any diseases that can be said to be supramental in origin as such with maybe one exception, depression. Depression happens due to lack of satisfaction in a long-time scale, a lack of involvement with the archetypes will do it. Depression can lead to physical symptoms as well.

Our lack of ongoing connection to the supramental and bliss bodies manifests as the ignorance that is the root cause of all suffering. The East

Indian sage Patanjali has said that ignorance gives rise to the ego, the ego develops likes and dislikes (a process we call mentalization of feeling), and these likes and dislikes eventually give rise to physical disease and fear of death.

Thus, physical disease can be caused at all the levels at which we live, at each of our five bodies. The strict materialist assumes that all disease is caused at the physical level and there is the most profound mistake of conventional medicine. But the alternate healing professionals make the same mistake if they attribute disease to any one level, as due to malfunction at any one body. In many cases, one must examine the cause of disease at more than one level.

Take the case of a physical injury. Materialists think that this is a physical-level problem. But after surgery, the wound does not heal. Now is the time to realize that the vital programs that assist the regeneration at the wound in the affected organ are not working properly. This is the time to consult an acupuncturist.

The same consideration holds for healing of all disease, which must also take place at more than one level. A disease comes with certain symptoms at the physical level, certain feelings of illness at the vital level, certain wrongness of meaning at the mental level, and a certain sense of separateness for the supramental and bliss levels. A complete healing is holistic healing—we should always try a multilevel approach, if a compatible approach can be found at the different levels.

Here is how it works. At the lowest level is conventional medicine and its materialist cures: drugs, surgery, and radiation. If the disease is entirely physical (which is seldom the case), then a material cure is the end of the story.

At the next level, the vital level, the disease has recognizable vital components as well as the obvious physical ones. If we treat only the vital components of the disease, as the Eastern practitioners of Ayurveda and Traditional Chinese Medicine do or as the homeopaths tend to do also, we have an exclusive paradigm. It is true that the treatment at the vital level is more fundamental and encompasses the physical level, but it takes time. It is also true that in some cases, when there is an urgency, the complementary use of the physical cure is clearly called for. The point is to focus on the compatibility of the two cures; then everything is in the right direction.

At the next level, the role of the mind is recognized, and this level is now that of mind-body disease and mind-body healing. Yes, at this level, the mind can be said to create the disease, but is it necessary to insist that mind alone heals: Is it all mind doing the healing at the mental level with that healing percolating down to the physical? Instead, why not continue compatible vital level and physical level healing as well?

In fact, mind-body healing is often a misnomer. When the mind creates the disease, often, the healing cannot be found at the level of the mind. One has to take a quantum leap to the supramental for healing. Of course, supramental healing does not exclude the mind; neither does it exclude the vital. A leap to the supramental fixes the wrongness of mental meaning; fixing the mental meaning fixes the vital feeling signifying the healing of the vital software reactivating the biological functions of the organs at the physical level. But of course, a leap to the supramental also can simultaneously lead to new mental meaning and mend the vital software as well.

At the next level of spiritual healing is the recovery of wholeness (etymologically healing and whole came from the same root). It can be reached in three different ways:

1. through situational healing of a particular dichotomy; or
2. through the fundamental realization of the archetype of wholeness; or
3. through what spiritual traditions call enlightenment.

Some confusion may arise regarding spiritual enlightenment. For instance, if spiritual enlightenment is also the highest level of healing, why do supposedly enlightened people die of disease such as cancer (so much so that the physician Andrew Weil jokingly calls enlightenment an invitation to cancer)? It is a fact that two great enlightened mystics of fairly recent times, Ramakrishna and Ramana Maharshi, both died of cancer. But this confusion dissolves when we recognize that the discovery of wholeness heals the mind of the ego-separateness, the healing of the ego gets rid of vital imbalances due to emotional preferences; no emotional preference means no fear of death at the physical level. So there is nobody there either to suffer or be afraid of death due to the disease. Who, then, needs to heal it? In other words, the enlightened perspective may not make sense to perspectives from any of the lower levels.

Why would disease come to enlightened people in the first place? Old-fashioned spiritual explorers put the body in enormous hardship with malnourishment, for example. It could also be genetic predisposition or past life's karma for these people.

QUANTUM INTEGRATIVE MEDICINE IN A NUTSHELL

Quantum Integrative Medicine consists of the following modus operandi:

- Quantum Integrative Medicine is based on a paradigm that most diseases occur simultaneously at more than one of the five bodies of consciousness: physical, vital, mental, supramental, and spiritual. However, the disease may originate in one level and spread to other levels from there.
- The goal of Quantum Integrative Medicine is not to treat disease by targeting one level (the material) as in allopathy, but to target all the movements of all five bodies of consciousness as the field of healing as necessary.
- Specifically, both the mind and vital energies are accepted as places where disease can originate and healing may take place.

Healing at a higher plane of consciousness heals the lower planes automatically, albeit taking time.
- Naturally, the crude and invasive techniques of physical body medicine, at least in part, must give way to subtler techniques.
- Illness and disease are clearly distinguished.
- The idea of self-healing is accepted as part of the potency of downward causation of consciousness. Other healing is accommodated as examples of nonlocality (see later).
- Physicians, therefore, once again, become cohealers along with the patient (see later).
- Preventive medicine, maintenance of well-being, is considered paramount.

You can see that many of these ideas are already being practiced in alternative medicine schools such as naturopathy. What is new here is quantum thinking, a conscious application of quantum principles to develop a thorough and workable scientific system of holistic healing that integrates all previous disparate systems of healing.

Practitioners of conventional medicine may still hesitate to embrace an integrative medicine that integrates alternative medicine with conventional medicine. If medicine were generalized to involve nonphysical domains of reality (even conceding that they exist), would medicine still be a science? Science depends on consensus experimental data. Since by definition we cannot observe the nonphysical directly with our physical instruments, how can we build a consensus science?

The answer to this kind of concern is now clear. Our individualized nonphysical bodies, the vital and the mental, are not susceptible to direct physical measurements, true, but they have correlated effects in the physical which are available for laboratory experimentation. Examples are Kirlian photography and biophoton emission tomography for the vital and fMRI for the mental. Moreover, we as conscious beings can directly feel, think, and intuit, which are our direct connections to the vital, the mental, and the supramental. Quantum physics demands that the doctrine of strong objectivity, namely, that science should be independent of subjects, is replaced by a doctrine of weak objectivity, namely, that science should be invariant from subject to subject. In this way, Quantum Integrative Medicine is weakly objective and therefore scientific.

chapter two

KNOW THY SELF, OH, QUANTUM DOCTOR

We heard this joke from a physician's assistant: A doctor dies and goes to heaven. To his surprise, he finds there is a long queue at the Pearly Gates. But of course, this doctor is not used to standing in a queue, so he goes right up to the front of the queue, expecting to be admitted immediately. When St. Peter stops him, the doctor is incensed. But St. Peter is firm, "Sorry, doctor. In heaven, even doctors have to learn to wait." Just at that moment a man in a long white coat with a stethoscope hanging from his neck goes running past, right through the gate.

"There goes another doctor," the doctor yells at St. Peter. "You let him in! That's not fair!" St. Peter chuckles. "Oh, that's God. Sometimes He thinks He's a doctor."

It's a joke and so we laugh. But it is also a tragedy because a doctor's ego-inflation closes his mind to the many things that we are talking about, namely, consciousness and the subtle objects of the world—vital energy, mental meaning, archetypal values—that play an essential role in healing.

If a doctor wants to be a healer, she or he has to transform and develop empathy. Becoming a doctor begins with presupposing that there is an "I" experience for everybody, not just her. Hers is inflated, and she needs to transform that. Then she has to confront her worldview anachronism of materialist science: How can everyone else be robots with experience but she is exempt from the rule? Not only does she have to presuppose "I," but she has to presuppose a causally potent "I" that uses its causal potency to change. Additionally, if a doctor wants to encourage his or her clients to take responsibility for their disease, healing, quality of life, etc., the patient's "I" also needs to be validated in order for the patient to change.

The belief in the West that there is no subject or self goes back to the days of Rene Descartes, who famously wrote, "I think, therefore I am," identifying "I," the self, as a part of the mind. The mind, of course, consists of thoughts—clearly objects. So the self is looked upon as a mental object, another thought. With subjective connotation, but so what? Call it subjective *qualia* and make it sound like an object. In this way, any question of causal potency of the self can also be avoided.

To make things even more interesting, there is indeed an object "me" that we mentally experience. Upon close inspection, "me" turns out to be an objectified version of the subject "I." In our ordinary experience of the "I," we do have the tendency of confusing between "I" and this "me." In ordinary experiencing, what we experience is I/me; we call this the ego. The ego has character, a conditioned pattern of habits and learning, as well as a persona, a sort of a head honcho like the CPU of learned programs.

How to experience the pure "I?" If we experience it, the prejudice—there is no subject/self, there are only objects—just falls away. Before we go into that, however, it is important to grasp how quantum physics deals with the problem of the self and causal power.

SUBJECT/SELF IN QUANTUM PHYSICS

To understand how the self-identity arises, we need to go into the quantum measurement problem, how quantum possibilities become objects of actuality. The physicist John von Neumann enunciated an observer effect: Without the observer there is no actualization of quantum possibilities. And that is only because an observer has something that is clearly nonmaterial, clearly outside the jurisdiction of quantum possibility math.

What must that be, this nonmaterial entity? Von Neumann referred to it vaguely as consciousness. What he meant is that the observer's conscious awareness of the subject-pole of experience which cannot be reduced to a bunch of objects, be they neurons of the brain. Following von Neumann's line of thinking—and there really is no other way to avoid paradox—the problem of quantum measurement must be seen as how the potential unity of the domain of potentiality splits into a subject (the "I" behind the eye of the brain) looking at an object (say, an electron plus the amplifying apparatus we use to look at the electron, such as a Geiger counter).

To repeat, the chain of logic should be clear: There is no other way to solve the measurement problem than via the observer effect. This means the oneness of the domain of potentiality splits into a subject-object polarity as an effect of quantum measurement. The subject is consciously aware of itself looking at the object.

In sum, in a quantum measurement, one consciousness splits into a subject and an object.

A TANGLED HIERARCHY IN THE BRAIN

The real problem to solve then is, how does the brain become the vehicle of the self or subject of the experience of the object? This is the hard question that has been answered in Amit's *The Self-Aware Universe*.

After actualization, consciousness is found to have identified with the brain and become the manifest observer who hears the tick of the electron at the Geiger counter and reports in the first person, "I hear the tick." The brain must be special to capture consciousness in this way. This special thing in the brain is called a tangled hierarchy: A tangle of two brain apparatuses that is able to capture consciousness as it uses the brain to look through it.

In a simple hierarchy, one level has causal power over the other in a linear relationship. A tangled hierarchy is a circular relationship, with each level creating the other, so you cannot tell which is at the top. It's like trying to answer the chicken-or-egg question: Which comes first?

How does a tangled hierarchy give self-identity? Following Doug Hofstadter (in his book, *Goedel, Escher, Bach*), consider the liar's sentence, "I am a liar." In an ordinary sentence, which you can recognize as a simple hierarchy, a sentence such as "I am an author," the predicate "author" qualifies the subject "I" once and for all. But notice the circularity of the liar's sentence: the predicate at the end qualifies the subject, but then a contradiction occurs, drawing our attention back to the beginning. If I am a liar, then I am telling the truth; and this goes on and on: If I am telling the truth then I am a liar, then I am telling the truth, ad infinitum.

If you enter the circularity of the sentence and identify with the circularity, you tend to get caught. Try it; you will think you are embodied in the sentence. Of course, in this case, it is easy for you to get out. After all, it is your tacit acceptance of the rules of the English grammar that got you involved also got you a self-identity. Technically speaking, you belong to the "inviolate" level of the implicit English grammar where the sentence cannot go, but you can. So you can get yourself in, and you can also get yourself out.

If the brain has a tangled hierarchical system within it, then when consciousness looks at objects through it, and chooses from the available quantum possibilities, it gets caught; the choice actualizes a brain state as well as the states of the objects. However, consciousness identifies with the brain and considers itself separate from the other actualized objects such as the Geiger counter and the electron. The observing subject/self—this is the present-centered quantum self—and the observed objects coarise in awareness via quantum actualization.

It works. In all events of perception, the perceiver's brain is always one of the objects involved, but the observer never experiences the brain separate from self. The experiencing brain and the self are like painting and canvas. You cannot peel one away from the other.

In the case of the liar's sentence, we really belong to the inviolate level, so the identification with the sentence is pretend identification; we can get off from identifying with the sentence at will. In the case of the brain, the inviolate level is our unconscious, we in ordinary ego cannot go there and retain our separateness and awareness and therefore our identification with the brain in manifest experience seems to be total; we cannot get out of the identification by wishing it or by virtue of this knowledge of the mechanism behind our identification. We gain something, a separate self, and that's huge. But we also lose something: we develop an ignorance of who we are, a kind of forgetfulness.

Here's an important question: Can we get out of our brain-identity from the quantum self? When we experience the quantum self in an intuitive or creative experience, we are so concentrated on the object of the experience, we obviously don't. But don't jump to conclusions yet. The great Buddha first explicitly reported, and there have been many confirmations ever since, that in a present-centered quantum self-experience if we pay attention to the self, we discover that it is really a no-self, and at that moment we really can choose to get out of the immanent manifest world and merge into the unconscious unity. (For more on this, see Amit's book *See the World as a Five-Layered Cake*.)

Back to the liar's sentence. The liar's sentence has two levels to make the tangle—the subject and the predicate; what are the two levels of the tangled hierarchy of the brain? Perception and memory are the dual partners of the brain's tangled hierarchy: There is no memory without perception; there is no perception without memory.

Pretend that you are entering the tangle with the idea of choosing and actualizing. Where do you start? Let's say you start with the perception apparatus. But that won't do; manifest perception requires manifest memory to be operational. So you shift attention to memory and try actualizing that. But that does not work either; there is no manifest perception to memorize. So you get caught in the brain going back and forth between the two apparatuses. The brain, because of its tangled hierarchy has acquired a self that sees itself separate from any other objects of perception.

What is really the case is this: 1) consciousness, the ground of the unconscious domain of potentiality actualizes both perception and memory apparatuses; 2) unconscious is the inviolate level and "you" can go there but so does the brain with you and both become potentiality; and 3) actualization is nonlocal.

All fit. In truth, perception and memory are made manifest both at the same fell-swoop by the act of downward causation causing the appearance of memory creating perception and perception creating memory.

Also, in the final reckoning, do not forget that like the Escher picture of *Drawing Hands* (Figure 5a), the brain's tangled hierarchy of its perception and memory apparatuses (Figure 5b), self-making and separateness are appearances, but they are by no means trivial. Consciousness creates these appearances in order to split itself into two parts: one part looking at the other as separate from itself.

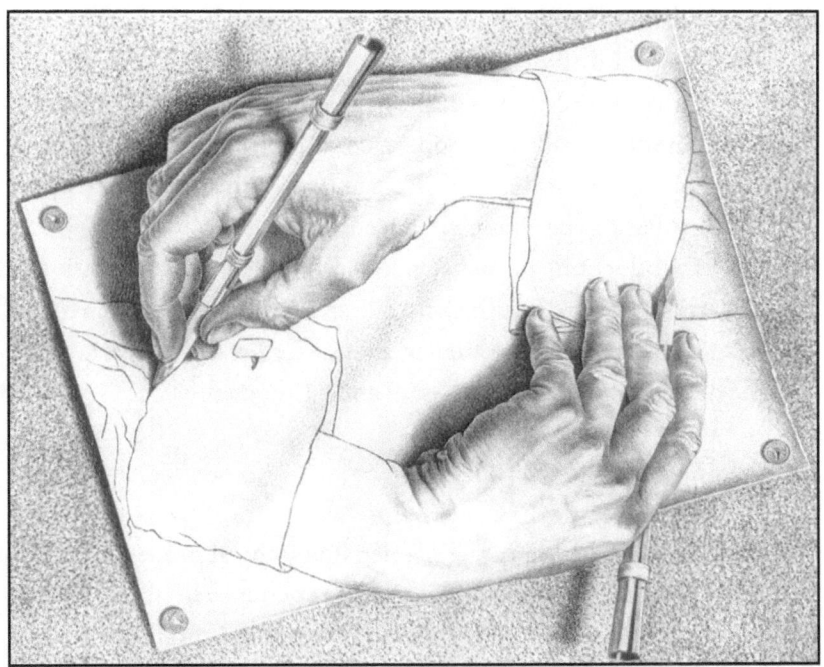

Figure 5a. Drawing Hands *by M.C. Escher (artist's rendition).*

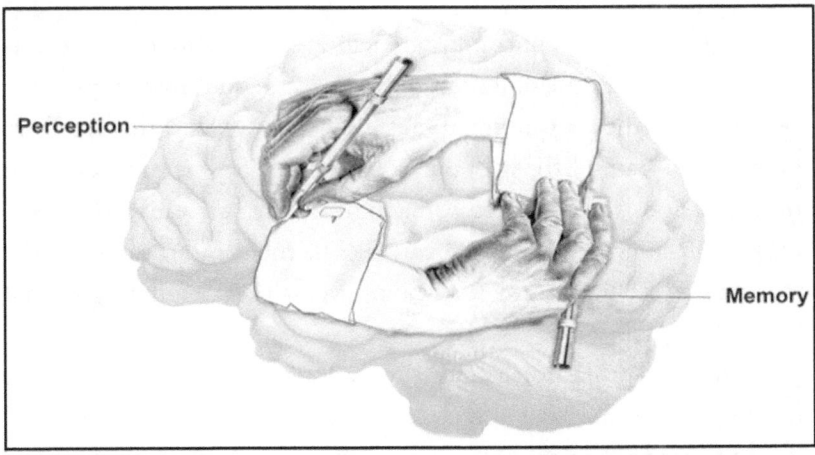

Figure 5b. The perception and memory apparatuses' tangled hierarchy, like Escher's hand, creates the appearance of circularity and self-identity.

Finally, because the separateness of the quantum self is not enough to produce the kind of forgetfulness we need for a stable manifest world experience, there is the process of subsequent reflection in the mirror of memory (Buddhists call it dependent coarising) before we experience the self in our ego. Neuroscientists have measured the time taken for the memory feedback to be about half a second.

In the introduction, we mentioned recent data that is revolutionizing our outlook toward health and healing. It is not only at the neocortex that we have tangled hierarchies; they also exist at the heart chakra and the navel chakra. (See Chapters 9 and 11 for details.)

THERE IS A SELF BEYOND THE EGO

The experience of the self of the tangled hierarchical processing in the brain, the subject of a subject-object split experience in its immediacy is always fresh; there is no prior memory of it. It has no individuality, it is cosmic. This is why we call it the quantum self. The Sanskrit word for this experience is *samadhi*. Intuition is a glimpse at the quantum self.

The quantum self is unconditioned, forever new, and it is what spiritual traditions call the inner self or higher self and transpersonal psychologists call the transpersonal self. If we move toward this self from the ordinary state of the ego, our consciousness seems expanded and this expansion is experienced as happiness. The subtle experiences—thinking, feeling, intuiting—all can take us there. Who can deny the importance of being happy for healing when we are suffering from a disease?

The medical profession is gradually acknowledging the value of music therapy, art therapy, meditation, etc. All these things work because they are happiness producing and take us toward the quantum self.

Your ordinary ego-experience is besought with "me," the objectified part of the I-experience. But, in contrast, the quantum self has no "me." It is a pure I-experience. Now the adage, "Physician, know thyself," makes sense, doesn't it? The self that is being referred to here is the quantum self. Physicians become healers when they explore the archetype of wholeness. These explorations lead to the discovery of the quantum self. A connoisseur of wholeness also is a master of empathy, and empathy is the ultimate goal of a healer—it is why you chose healing as your profession.

If you bring the quantum worldview to your healing profession and at the same time continue to explore the archetype of wholeness to discover your true self, you are a quantum doctor, a quantum healer.

Now you must see why we have provided all these details about the tangled hierarchy. Dear healer, to develop empathy and a nonlocal connectedness with your client you need to give up simple hierarchical behavior toward your client and practice tangled hierarchy instead.

THE EGO

We have begun to examine how the ego arises from our initial quantum-self response to every external stimulus via dependent coarising. Now, let's elaborate on that.

Every time the memory apparatus of the tangled hierarchy finishes processing any stimulus, it makes a memory of the stimulus-response. When the same stimulus arrives at the brain, the memory plays back giving a secondary stimulus, a reflected image so to speak. So the quantum perception system has to respond not only to the primary stimulus but also the secondary stimulus. You can think of this processing of feedback as a reflection in the mirror of memory. It biases the system to respond in favor of the previous response. In this way, many such reflections produce what psychologists call conditioning.

When reflecting on memory, we each also see ourselves experiencing a me. The more we undertake memory reflection, the greater the me-experience; gradually, the experience of "I" becomes implicit, more like, "I am this me." We also develop personality programs, and we choose our response depending on the situation. This finally makes us into a simple hierarchical ego/persona—the head honcho of our personality programs.

THE QUESTION OF FREE WILL

Initially, for the quantum self, the conscious choice that creates experience presents infinite potentialities from which to choose. Having more and more memory accumulation for identical stimuli and more and more conditioning, under slightly different environmental situations, produces conditioning with a more limited spectrum of choices. The system is still quantum, but the feedback has limited the conscious freedom to choose at the ego level. In this way, the ego has free will, but with a limited conditioned spectrum of choice.

Likewise, the feelings coupled with sensing or with thought that the ego chooses in response to a stimulus—the vital software—are conditioned within this limited spectrum of choice. For the vital, this leaves room for situational adjustment to a stimulus-response, something avant-garde physicians call the body's wisdom. However, the body needs a clear indication of what the ego wants; so, ultimately, it is still the choice of the ego.

FROM THE EGO TO THE QUANTUM SELF: THE THREE QUANTUM PRINCIPLES

Free choice, an act of downward causation, ultimately resides in the unconscious; however, the signature that we have chosen freely is found in the quantum-self experience in this form: "I did not have this experience via rational thinking." In this way, the closer we learn to live in the expanded consciousness of the quantum self, the easier it is for us to access the source of free choice.

Downward causation—free choice of Oneness consciousness—comes to us in three ways: nonlocality, discontinuity, and tangled hierarchy. These are the ways we reconnect to the quantum self and real freedom.

Nonlocality is communication without signals, instead of signals using nonlocal consciousness for communication. There is a catch, however. To use nonlocality with another, you two have to correlate, activate your potential oneness. This correlation can be done easily via positive interaction, meditation with intention, or simply strong intention.

Patients who recuperate from surgery intend to heal quickly, no doubt, but due to their special situation, they may live a little far away from the quantum self. Can their healing intention be augmented through intention and prayer by another even from a distance, using nonlocality? The answer is yes. This phenomenon is called distance healing, which physician Randolph Byrd first demonstrated in 1988. Several patients at a hospital in San Francisco were recuperating from cardiac surgery. Byrd gave a list of the patients to a prayer group in another city far away. The prayer group chose names from the list at random and did their intentions and prayers all double blind. Neither Byrd nor the patients knew who exactly was prayed for. But there was an improvement in healing rates for the people who were being prayed for, which went way beyond what could be expected from random statistical fluctuations of the healing rate. Admittedly, there is controversy about distance-healing experiments, and there are many articles that refute Byrd's. However the researcher Jeanne Achterberg did a very thorough conclusive experiment which should settle the issue.

This is only one kind of use of nonlocality in healing. More telling are the studies—one of which was published in the *JAMA [Journal of American Medical Association] Internal Medicine* in 2016 and mentioned in *Time* magazine's February 26, 2018 issue—showing that people who regularly go to church and worship with a group of other people live longer and healthier lives. Is their longevity due to being church members and following a religion? Not necessarily. It may be activated nonlocality and unity consciousness that brings people a sense of happiness that promotes their health.

This is why empathy on the part of the healer is so important for healing, for what is empathy but the ability of maintaining a nonlocal connection with another person for prolonged periods at a time which spiritual traditions call opening the heart to include others (Figure 6). How else would a healer be in the client's shoes, feel the suffering of the other, and let go of it when the need for connection is over?

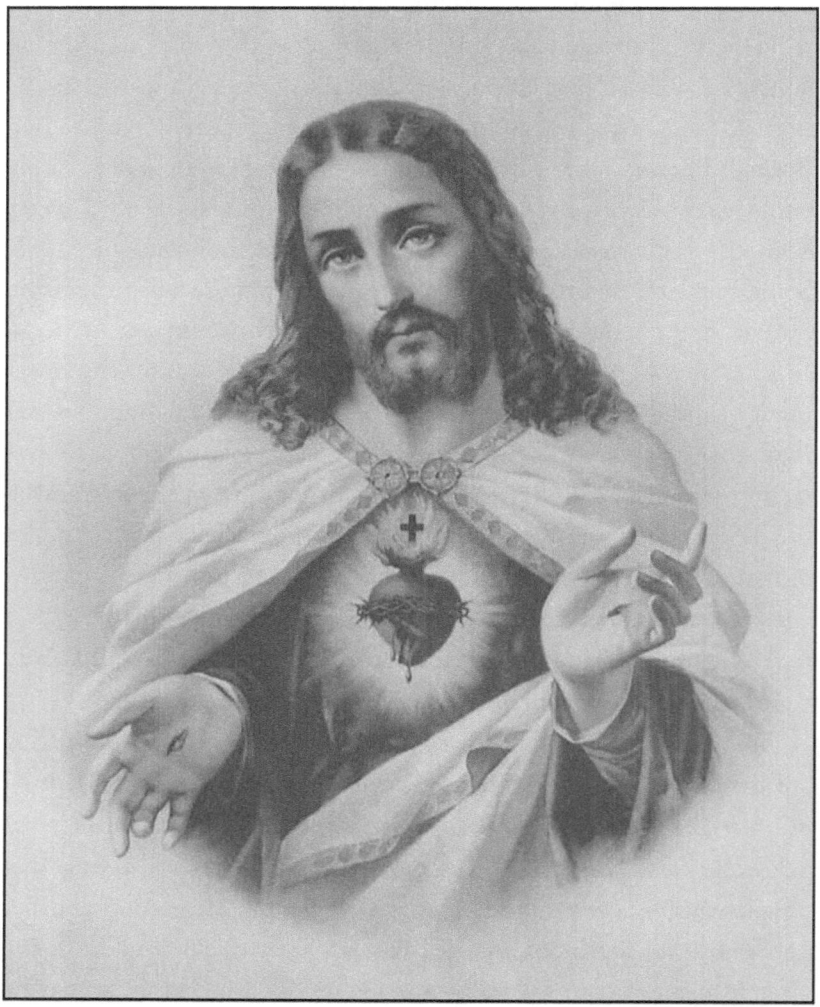

Figure 6. People who are empathetic, like Jesus, have an expanded heart.

Discontinuity is a jump between places that are not continuously connected by a bridge. When electrons jump from one atomic orbit to another, they do not go through the intervening space; instead, they take what is said to be a discontinuous quantum leap (Figure 7).

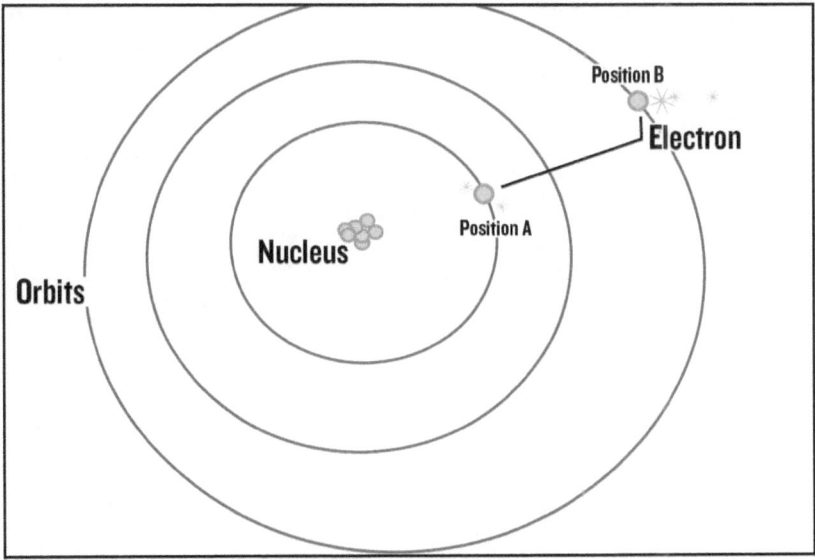

Figure 7. A quantum leap, as envisioned by Niels Bohr, who posits that when electrons jump from one atomic orbit to another, they never go through the intervening space. Many experiments support Bohr's theory.

Earlier, we mentioned spontaneous healing without medical intervention. The physician Deepak Chopra has theorized that such healings are due to quantum leaps. A wrong mental meaning given to a stimulus causes a vital energy block at a vital organ that eventually translates into the physical disease of the correlated physical organ. When the patient takes a quantum leap in thought correcting the mental meaning, the energy block is spontaneously removed and she is healed without any continuous medical intervention—quantum healing.

Thus, looking at health and healing through the worldview of quantum physics immediately endows the healer and the patient with the power of downward causation, with the potential power of choosing health over disease. What remains is to learn the subtleties of the exercise of this choice. And when you do, you find out why such self-healing is traditionally called a healing by a higher power, Spirit or God: because it takes you out of your ordinary separate cocoon of existence to a holistic, nonlocal level of being.

chapter three

PREVENTION: A NEW AND ESSENTIAL PERSPECTIVE

In the Bhagavad-Gita, Krishna says: "Learn to fully know the ultimate center of your being. The one that is mysterious, indestructible and transcendent. The immortal transcendental Self, *Atman*, which exists in every human being. Nobody was ever able to destroy or to disturb this spirit that exists in every being."

When Jacques Parre, who invented the first element of surgery, was becoming famous for saving soldiers on the battlefield with his surgical operations, he would say about each patient who survived, "I treated him, but God healed him."

Paracelsus, the great healer and alchemist, said: "God had been providing all that is needed to the human being to be cured. The role of science is to find it. The art of healing starts in nature and one should look in nature to learn."

Also, there is a popular saying: "There is an herb for any disease. You only have to find it."

In these modern times, many people are asking themselves: "Is it possible to cure a disease by methods different from conventional medicine, methods that really heal both the underlying cause and symptoms, methods without side effect, methods that do not compromise quality of life?"

Our world today is, for many of us, full of suffering, and the methods which efficiently heal, not just cure the symptoms of new diseases are facing a very big challenge from not only the medicine establishment but also from the culture. More and more people are looking for a state of harmony and balance in their lives—they seek happiness but their quest for harmony and happiness seems to be constantly thwarted. Of course, many individuals are hit by different individual kinds of problems, but there is one common thread: People are in a hurry. Methods for authentic healing do not work that way.

When I (Valentina) look at the history of modern medicine, I notice that history exemplifies the Greek story of Sisyphus—the man who would roll a stone uphill until he reached the top, only to have the stone fall back down on him, over and over again. Sisyphus was doomed to this punishment due to some mistakes he had made. To me, this is a metaphor for what is happening in modern medicine. Each time modern medicine successfully cures or finds a method to cure or diminish the influence of a disease, another disease comes into the picture. I maintain that today there are many new diseases that people suffer that did not exist before.

The medicine establishment objects to this. They say that, in fact, people's awareness is growing and therefore we have become aware of many more diseases that haunt us today, unlike in the previous times when this awareness was lacking.

An often used example is diabetes. Diabetes is a disease of which people were aware of in ancient times, but there were no sure-fire methods to diagnose diabetes until recently. The only diagnostic method for diabetes in antiquity which I have ever heard about was the "bee test." A person suspected of having diabetes had to pee into a bowl. That bowl was placed next to another bowl containing the urine of a normal person. Theoretically, the bees would be attracted to the urine of the diabetic person because it was very sweet compared with the other urine since a normal person's pancreas is able to process sugar while the diabetic one expels it unprocessed.

Doesn't it seem obvious that though there were many people dying of diabetes in ancient times, the statistics of diabetes were not available until the twentieth-century medical profession began creating and perpetuating a misinformation?

As the meditation teacher Advaitananda emphasized in a lecture on health that I (Valentina) attended years ago, there is a principle in nature: Every phenomenon that exists does so because it is needed. However, there is a corollary, which is that whatever people intend and focus on, if the intention is archetypal, it manifests. In antiquity, in terms of health, the culture was focused on the archetype of wholeness, and whether people manifested it. Doctors were paid only until the patients remained healthy; people stopped paying the doctor when they got ill and the doctor had to treat them for free.

In contrast, these days we mainly focus on diseases. We don't look at the status of our health, let alone take good care of our health, unless disease hits us. When we have a disease, we call it by a name, we make it into an enemy and fight against it, and we even turn the entire society to fight a crusade. Our main focus is upon disease, not upon health. We don't want to maintain health or to have that as our crusade; instead, we try to keep the focus on disease.

Of course, we cannot back up every claim about the past, but that is not the objective of this discussion. The fact is, we now have a scientific theory that confirms the old belief that health is balance and harmony, while disease is imbalance and disharmony. It's important to realize that you cannot avoid the imbalance unless you focus on the balance. The imbalance begins as we stop growing, and as we get older. This is the root of our current health crisis, which mostly involves middle-aged and older people. The situation which we face nowadays in the whole medical system and in the whole health industry is that we look at the problem from the wrong end. More balanced thinking is needed.

While optimistic people focus on the source of light, pessimists and cynics focus on the shadows cast. This is the reason why we cannot even take "miraculous" healings seriously; we assume that, maybe at best, it was a coincidence. When we try to replace the miracle with a coincidence, by having this attitude, we try to create a world in which healing miracles are not possible. When, in the 1980s we started paying attention to the data without doubting its veracity, we discovered the science of these miracles—quantum healing. Today, we fully understand how quantum healing works and people are healing themselves by following quantum healing's quite scientific procedure.

These days more and more scientists are demonstrating the impact that our mind and imagination have upon the physical world. We create our own world with our own concepts, with the principles we think and live by. But the way we see problems is the problem. Therefore, when we speak about maintaining or optimizing (healing) the status of health of a human being, we have to understand and know by direct experience what health is. Then we will be able to maintain the status of health or improve upon it. As long as we are only aware when something is painful, and as long as we are aware when something is disturbed or unbalanced at the physical, emotional, or mental level, we will only know consciously examples of disease and its symptoms. Then how can we take care of our own health, let alone help somebody keep health when they don't have a clue about what it is?

Here is an example from Advaitananda. Suppose you go to a person who is extremely ill and you tell that person: "Try to be healthy," The person will say, "How? It's extremely painful. Help me relieve the pain!" The person is only aware of the pain. Once you give someone a painkiller, that person will consider himself or herself cured, and will never focus upon the fact that they are now healthy. The person is not going to rejoice, "Look how healthy I am, look how harmonious I am. Look how well I feel in this moment. I should remember this wellness. I should try to maintain it."

So, because of our unawareness of ourselves, when we are disturbed, we become aware of what we are not. We become aware of particular cases of disease and suffering. We become aware of imbalances, and for this reason what happens goes something like this: While people are young their status of health goes up and down in a rhythm which is manageable by the body's built-in system. Young people abuse their own bodies and their own minds by doing all kinds of risky things. The human being is designed in such a wonderful way that it has a lot of reserves in software; so therefore, when we are young, we can go out a lot and overdo everything, yet our body can manage to compensate for our mistakes and get back on the track. Eventually though, when our body and mind are overloaded by the mistakes we have made and one more mistake happens, and the system cannot compensate and from that moment on, according to studies and doctors' observations, people actually never recover in full. Instead, they develop a state of permanent imbalances. This is called the *prakriti* (a combination of doshas) of their physical-vital system.

People start the healing journey from a place of disease; when they recover a little bit, they go to another problem, another mistake, another disease. Again, they recover a bit, then go create another problem and another disease and slowly this imbalance continues until the status of health is severely damaged and they go out of the game, so to speak, when they die. This is usually the pattern which people who get ill follow to their old age. After one severe disease, we never truly recover. We recover somewhat though, and mistake it for a return of health; so, when the doctor asks, "Do you still have pain?" we say no. But if we truly knew what health is, we would be more sensitive and see that the condition still is not quite there in balance to call it good health. If I cannot tell that I'm different than I was before and that not being the same will add to another experience of not being the same, slowly but surely, and also faster and faster, my status of health will decay, because in fact I don't know how to recover or what complete recovery feels like.

Most people don't remember how it is to be healthy; therefore, the first condition to recover before we begin to talk with our clients more deeply about all these aspects of disease and health, is to understand that our approach to this subject should drastically be re-visioned, and radically put right side up, because otherwise, no matter what we say about health, we're talking about something which the clients don't know any more.

A real scientist is a person who is open in his mind and in his heart for what is new. A real scientist is open to miracles, and he accepts each miracle as a temporary hypothesis for his exploration. A false scientist is a professional skeptic who will just reject the facts.

Now, thanks to quantum physics, there is another aspect of us which we are invited to be aware of as we begin our journey toward health: In virtually every spiritual text, we find, one way or another, references to the immortal spirit of every being. This spirit exists beyond all conflicts, being permanently present as a witness, observing with equanimity our mistakes as well as our righteous actions, our aging as well as our youth, our suffering as well as our pleasure, our death as well as our life. This is Quantum reality within, and it should be seriously taken in any discussion about healing.

Quantum reality means that every human being deep inside, in the ultimate essence of potentiality, is perfect, harmonious, balanced, capable of manifesting all the attributes of perfection. But due to some, let's say, processes of ignorance or mistakes (some of it due to the nature of evolution), we arrive at particular cases when we consider ourselves disturbed, ill, unbalanced, unlucky, or unhappy—or we fall dead. So, the first step in any process of healing is to restore this understanding, this vision.

Consider once again that in nature, nothing appears if it is not needed. But how about happiness: Do you think that happiness (expanded consciousness) appears without having any meaning? If you think so, if you don't feel any need for it, it will disappear. If you don't find any use for it, it will disappear. If you don't find any use for your memory, it will disappear. If you don't find any use for your life, that will gradually disappear too. But first life will give you some signs—the first sign is suffering of some kind, followed by greater suffering in more varieties and less quality of life, and gradually, one day, life will tend to disappear altogether. And then you are confronted with the process of death. This will not happen only once, this will happen every time you fail to explore the meaning or purpose of your life. This is the fundamental law of nature: For everything we experience in this life, if it doesn't have a meaning for us, it will disappear.

It is very interesting how people's minds react to all of this. We can easily understand these things if we look at the entire culture and how it behaves. Even the modern physical scientist, upon studying the universe, is reluctantly reaching the same conclusion: The universe itself evolves so that life is created, so that sentience can come about. This is called the anthropic principle: The universe has a purpose. Why sentience? The psychologist Carl Jung said that the purpose of consciousness is to make the unconscious conscious. Why does consciousness want to do that? The biologist and theologian Teilhard de Chardin said consciousness wants to see its infinite possibilities explored, lived, and embodied; in this way, we create heaven on this very earth. Exploring meaning and purpose is what we are here for, and this is the key to health, prosperity, and happiness.

Everything which happens in our life has a certain meaning and purpose—and realizing that is the first step in our process of healing, spiritual healing. What will be that meaning? What will be the sense, the purposive direction our life follows? Basically, all the books of wisdom, in talking about the status of health, don't talk about diseased people; instead, they talk about health, harmony, happiness—they say the same thing as de Chardin, that the purpose of life is to explore the infinite possibilities that consciousness has given us to explore.

It's very interesting, isn't it? On the one hand, the wisdom traditions have discovered who we truly are and they say we are potentially perfect, we are extraordinary, we are the manifestation of God and so on; on the other hand, they say that the purpose of our life is to explore and discover the many facets of God (the archetypes) and embody them. This is how health and harmony and happiness come to us. This is the reason why the people who wrote the wise books did not feel much need to write a manual about healing disease, because they believed the problem was solved by positing the problem in the right way. Instead, they developed healing science as Ayurveda: *Ayu* is a Sanskrit word meaning longevity, and *veda* is a Sanskrit word meaning creatively revealed knowledge of how to achieve longevity—a long life of health and happiness.

The way most people see the problem of health today is as the problem of curing disease. The problem was solved by the people of antiquity by positing the problem correctly. In this way, wise people in antiquity hardly talked about the detailed causes of disease and healing; in the main, they ascribed disease to one fundamental cause: ignorance.

Of course, in the here and now, our job as scientists of consciousness is cut out for us. We have to go further with our investigation and develop a proper science of health as preventive medicine. This book is a start in that direction. Simultaneously, we are attempting to help those who are ready to understand that our ignorance of the right way to think is basically creating all these problems we are subjected to in our daily life. Some of the ignorance manifests as mental illnesses, some as emotional stress, some eventually as physical illnesses.

Ignorance begins by ignoring our true nature that consciousness, not matter, is our ground of being; this is the first step of ignorance. Ignorance multiplies when we think we are just a physical body; by thinking we are our physical body, we interfere with its natural balance with correlated vital rhythms; when we interfere, the body's vital-physical duo starts to react. Ignorance multiplies when mind enters the game, when we precondition our status of happiness on things which exist outside of us via mental imagination, thus exposing ourselves to unhappiness of the unfulfillment of desires for pleasure. Realize that unhappiness, being just the shadow of happiness, doesn't exist as such. So, when we mistake the shadow as real object, we invite suffering.

In this way, we can see that illness is nothing else but a sign of imbalance or a sign of disorder trying to settle in. This illness, this state of disorder generates suffering and it is always born from our thoughts of wrong meaning that contract our consciousness—from materialistic visions of making temporary happiness permanent in the form of too much pleasure, from our uncontrolled desires stemming from negative emotions, and these negative aberrations of thoughts and emotions are in fact pushing away the beneficial and harmonizing positive influence of our heart. So all these things we carry with us as desires—as uncontrolled passions, as thoughts which are not in harmony with the universal laws—are just pushing away this beneficial influence which comes from our spirit via our heart. Therefore, we simply interfere with a process which is always self-regenerating, a self that is centered in happiness.

In antiquity, older people growing wiser was the norm; oh, those people were beautiful—they grew old, but they didn't suffer. Even in cases of proven diseases in their physical body, they didn't suffer much because they didn't identify with the suffering and remained expanded in consciousness, and happy; when they grew older they died peacefully, consciously. There were exceptions to be sure, but it is a fair guess that the wise people went through the experience of death in a conscious way.

What is the difference between the wise people of the old times and the people now? Well, the ones growing older and wiser in antiquity were paying attention to the status of their health; the ones growing older and suffering more and more now are focused on the status of disease, not health. Because of stopping the self-regenerative process which exists in all human beings who explore meaning and purpose, a regenerative process we call "soul-making" in the new science, as people today become old they degenerate into a soul-less life in which there is no living of new possibilities.

Traditionalists can argue about the increase of life expectancy but most of that is due to better hygiene, antibiotics, and improved surgery. These gains notwithstanding, we are pointing out further gains to be had with an attitudinal change.

Realize this: The quantum self, with its perfect radiance, is trying to impregnate all the structures in us—the soul, the mind, the vital, and the physical—creating new harmony, restoring harmony in the old, if we let it. If we block ourselves from this, the ego/personality turns into a narcissistic shell around the quantum self and doesn't allow its harmonizing radiance to take us through the process of regeneration. Self-healing is stopped and the process of aging becomes more and more difficult, more and more disharmonious and painful and so on. The main characteristic of this aging—Alzheimer's disease—is confusion. After a lifetime of struggle with ignorance, ending up in confusion is extremely difficult to manage.

Illness is just a necessary reminder for us to go back to the center, to return to dwelling on what is true in our being. It reminds us that we have lost our way. Exactly as when a person wanders into thorny bushes, the thorns in the bushes will pierce her skin, giving her a signal: Hey, you're off the road. If the woman is stupid, she will continue going the wrong way and hit some trees or something, making the situation worse; if she's even more stupid she will hit a rock or something; and so on, until she dies. Then she will come back into another life and again live for a little while traveling on the right road, and again will go off the road and again will receive signals: "Hey, that's wrong." This is how karma plays in our lives. The movie *Groundhog Day* provides an excellent rendition of the problem and the solution.

What is the solution? We should look upon these states of imbalance—disease—as the signals we get from Life and the Universe, showing us that we are breaking the laws of the science of consciousness and that we are not on the right path, which is supposed to be a path of increasing wholeness and happiness. The essence of the new paradigm of healing is that we must look upon the physical body as the material vehicle for the spirit to manifest. The physical organs are computer hardware. The rest of the parts of our bodies serve as software and causes and contexts of the software. From this perspective, the health problems, different disturbances of the perfect balance are only messages sent to us by the Spirit through the physical body in order to become aware of the level we have on the path of our journey of evolution and development.

PREVENTION

From this new perspective, the physical body is the mirror which helps us to see the state in which our spiritual life and state of happiness and well-being currently is. Therefore, any real healing process has to begin with learning the spiritual lesson of the illness we are confronted with and then graduate toward eliminating the cause which created the illness. With this change in perspective, we see disease for what it is—the absence of health—instead of seeing health as the absence of disease and getting lost in degenerative pursuits. Prevent the degeneration and you will never lose health; you'll never lose something you know and covet and you'll never stop paying attention. This, dear reader, is the essence of preventive medicine.

So take your first step right now. See a disease, any disease, as the obstacle to manifesting your potentialities of perfect health and happiness, and then make an intention: choose health, happiness, and wholeness.

chapter four

RESONANCE: THE SECRET OF BEING POSITIVE— AND THE EXPANDED CONSCIOUSNESS, WELLNESS, AND HAPPINESS THAT COME WITH IT

What is resonance? If you ask a physics teacher, she or he will hold up a tuning fork, strike the tuning fork with a little hammer and get it vibrating. The teacher will then hold the vibrating fork against his wooden desk; and you will notice that the desk is vibrating now, too. This is called forced vibration. The teacher will now hold up another tuning fork and get that one vibrating. But this time, when she or he touches the table with his vibrating fork, the table vibrates with much greater intensity. This is a resonance, a frequency matching. The table's natural frequency of vibration is matched by this fork's frequency of vibration.

Army engineers have had to learn this idea quickly. It was not infrequent that soldiers would march on a bridge and the bridge would collapse because the frequency of the marching matched the natural vibrational frequency of the bridge.

But still, this is physics. How does the concept of resonance apply to us in our daily lives? We have been talking about happiness as expansion of consciousness. Looking at a flower or a sunset may lead to an expansion of consciousness, which explains the exaltation you sometimes feel with such an experience. Even the intellectual Sigmund Freud talked about getting oceanic feelings. Why this expansion? Why are such experiences sometimes pleasant but ho-hum and other times oceanic?

Little expansions of consciousness often happen to us; we call them moments of relaxation. And then you look at a flower or a sunset in those special occasions, and whammo—a big expansion! We hope you understand this analogy: little expansions of consciousness are like forced vibration; big expansions exemplify the resonance phenomenon.

But what is resonating with what? What is vibrating in a flower that you can perceive? Is it sense perception we are talking about? This is where the physical scientists get lost. To them, such resonance talk is nonsense. There is no physical vibration in a flower that travels outside to us; nor does a body organ vibrate in a measurable way unless it has electrical components like the brain and the heart. However, new research with sound and music shows that there is some vibrating stuff in our body.

But of course, for us connoisseurs of consciousness, a flower is not only a material body—it is also alive, and it has vital software. The vital software is a representation of vital functions of archetypal origin, part of the laws of consciousness science, and the archetype of truth. The vital movements also guide the biological forms during evolution and development together, called "evo-devo." Through that guidance, consciousness injects the archetypes of beauty and wholeness in the natural world of plants.

I (Valentina) first discovered the concept of resonance in traditional yoga teachings, and immediately saw its direct application in both healing and transformation.

When an organ's evolved form and function match the intended archetypal biological form and function perfectly, the whole becomes greater than the parts, and the physical-vital reveals what some of us experience as beauty. Here, again, there are people who don't experience the beauty of a flower. To explain the difference in response, we use the concept of resonance.

What resonates with—what? Carl Jung discovered humanity's

collective unconscious in which the Platonic archetypes are represented as dichotomies of positive and negative: good versus evil, beauty versus ugly, truth versus lie, and so forth. When a stimulus—a sunset or a flower—evokes in us a positive experience of expansion of consciousness and increases the vital energy we feel and deepens the meaning we give to it, we call it a resonance: the stimulus we cognize is resonating with a positive archetype in our collective unconscious. Attention is crucial. If attention is lacking or the "frequency matching" between your cognition and the archetype is not exact, there is little expansion of consciousness and only minor appreciation of beauty. If you are inattentive, lost in your own conditioned thought, and unmindfully come up with only the socially correct response to the stimulus, "Oh, look at this beautiful flower," you may miss the beauty altogether.

This brings us to the concept of negative resonance—the evocation of a negative dual counterpart of an archetype. We think that a process of negative resonance—the absence of resonance due to inattention or callousness or worldview or belief system distortion—certainly exists in the experiential structure of a person who is having a disease. If we take the point of view of resonance here, it is mainly to look upon negative resonance rather than positive resonance. Somehow our wrong attitude might trigger that particular negative resonance, but no matter what we say about a disease, somewhere in our body it manifests as such a negative resonance that we experience an avoidance of resonance, a reluctance and inability to expand consciousness.

Of course, the sceptic in you may say, "Yeah, all right; if you have cancer, this makes some sense, but what if you break your leg? Where is the negative resonance there? Surely it is an external physical force that broke the bone." Well, you're right, it was a physical force that caused the break, but there may be something else involved, too. In some cases, the same attitude that led to your incapacity to appreciate beauty may also have led to the inattention that led you to break your leg.

Some psychologists may even go as far as to say that somewhere in your mindset are negative intentions. By your inattention they grow in intensity because whenever you are inattentive it is a fact that consciousness collapses your conditioned thoughts on an average probabilistic basis. So actually, somewhere in your mental history, you may have had a broken leg intention three months ago, but you didn't feel it, and that broken leg intention attracted like a magnet, through resonance, the events in your life. It is "aligning the stars," so to speak poetically, so that an event in which you'll break your leg or something like that will come there as potentiality and that is when you'll break your leg. It is not coming out of the blue with no warning signs. It is a negative resonance. Of course, the fact is that you should choose this extreme way of taking responsibility for disorders only when you are ready for it; otherwise, don't.

If negative intentions do us harm, the converse must also be true, positive intensions should do us good. This idea is popular with New Age people. Some people will say, "I understand that if I have a skin problem, I'll treat it with positive thoughts, but how can you treat a broken leg with positive thoughts?" Actually, if you don't treat it with positive thoughts you have immense chances that either you'll never recover, you'll get an infection, or you will have a lot of trouble from it, which will prove the fact that there is a negative resonance.

You New Age people should be clear too: Positive intentions and thoughts are only a start, not the end for the healing process. You have to follow up your positive intention with a creative process that will include the orthopedic surgeon who fixes up your bones and puts you in a plaster cast to keep the pieces immobile. If you engage in creatively continuing your healing intention during the long wait for getting the cast off, it will enhance the needed software to activate the function of regeneration. You will heal quickly. Your surgeon would love that. On the other hand, it is a fact that many broken bones don't heal so fast, so what gives? Negative intention. How it works can be found in the details of the creative process.

The creative process consists of four stages: preparation, unconscious processing achieved when we relax and quantum possibility waves of archetypes, meanings, and feelings can expand and grow producing new possibility, the quantum leap of insight when we choose a gestalt of actualities from all the possibilities, and finally manifestation—immediate change of the affected software to higher function followed by life style change as according to the new insight.

When healing from orthopedic surgery, the work of the surgeon and your emotional preparation for it is just the first stage; the long hiatus of keeping the plaster cast in place constitutes the second stage of unconscious processing. This is called "incubation" since you are doing nothing except sitting on your healing wound with healing intention the way a bird expectantly sits on her egg to hatch. Regeneration takes place at the onset of your healing insight, which is the moment at which the archetype of wholeness resonates with you. Manifestation, in this case, means to institute creativity and creative process in your belief system of how intentions work.

Okay, it is agreed that broken legs are usually healed via surgery and will not necessarily need your active participation. But how about healing cancer? Perhaps you can believe that the same creative process can affect your healing except for one modification: You have to alternate between preparation and incubation a few times like in that Frank Sinatra song—*do-be-do-be-do*. How hard can it be to maintain creative intention as you do-be-do-be-do with your doctor's help until that healing resonance takes place?

So, actually, there is always some resonance which is influencing your life as it is developing: good or bad, happy or unhappy, successful or unsuccessful, healthy or unhealthy. It is the process of resonance, positive or negative, that most affects us. We are always, no matter what else we are doing, in the process of ongoing possibilities of resonance with the archetypes in our lives—abundance, power, beauty, love etc. We tune in with different archetypes—positive resonance or not tune in at all—negative resonance. The melodrama begins when we forget it, when we are not aware of our negativity; sometimes we think the universe is turning off, the resonances are turned off, nobody is watching, so we can do whatever we want. But that's not true. No matter what we are doing, even when we are sleeping (yes, archetypes enter your dreams and when they do, you see them represented by the Jungian symbols or gods and goddesses of your culture), we are engaged in the ongoing process of resonance with the archetypes. Actually, we resonate on many levels at the same time, but we also have one that is the main resonance, and that one is ongoing.

Let's say someone says, "I want to have a happy life." I usually answer, "Good. What are you doing about it?"

"But I am not happy."

"Well, that's a consequence."

"What do you do about having a happy life?"

"How much attempt at happiness do you put in your life, so that you have it?"

"Well, I didn't think in that way..."

And this dialogue continues with people who come to me (Valentina) as clients.

Most of the time, I see that people, even people with a severe disease, don't apply the basic things they know to their life. For example, think of a person who is almost dying because of lung problems eating a lot of cheese and milk and all kind of dairy, and if I ask, "Do you know that this kind of things can kill you?" the person answers, "Yeah, of course, but they are so good..."

Even a healthy person eating too much milk products will be exposed to the possibility of all kinds of lung disfunctions.

To apply the law of resonance also means to learn about yourself and to learn what creates what resonance, but that's a process of observation; we have a built-in system of vital movements in our personal and collective unconscious, we just have to observe the feelings their movements generate. Once you observe that and get the hang of how to observe and be sensitive, you will know. The law of resonance requires only attention, nothing else. When you pay attention to the things you are doing and not doing and to the created expansion or contraction of consciousness because of the things you are doing, you will be amazed by how much of that is influencing your mood, the color of your face, or the tone of your voice. You will also be amazed how much the ongoing resonances of your lives are influencing the way you look, the way you hold your head and orient your shoulders, your attitude in life, and so on.

For example, if you have a problem with your lungs you will see that much of the time you will have the tendency to hold your palm next to your chest and stand in a crouching position. Guess why? Because, instinctively, your body is trying to preserve the heat in the chest area while your mind is trying to create a certain resonance.

You need to learn to analyze the whole environment you're living in; you'll see that, more often than not, you live in a "cold" environment with cold colors and no nourishing substances around you, and so on. You only have to be aware of this and you will know exactly what to change. Change colors, change your attitudes, change the temperature in your room, change a lot of things, and suddenly you will see that the disease is abating, often with no medicine. My experience is that it's around 70 percent chance that the disease will disappear just by your forming positive intentions and modifying the environment to a positive one. And to my surprise, recent research verified my estimate: about 70 percent of the cures by pharmaceutical drugs are actually "placebo cures," which is the name that the medical establishment has given to curing via positive intentions.

You can also boost your positive environmental effect quite a bit with some indoor plants and fresh flowers, of course (sorry, artificial flowers don't have much use), and in only about 30 percent of cases you will need a little bit more help from doctors and medicines, and that's it. We can get most of the problems we face in our lives to disappear just by working a little bit on the settings around us, because these settings determine to a large extent the resonances we have and the expansion (and contraction) of consciousness we create within our lives.

It's also very important to note here, of course, the food we eat and the air we breathe: the resonances created by the way we eat, the types of food we eat, the way we breathe, and the air we breathe. These two things: eating and breathing—nourishing ourselves—involve two of our major exchanges with the environment. So of course we can influence our being so much starting with the physical body.

There is the ancient saying: "You are what you eat." Expand this saying: "You are what you eat *and how you eat.*" If you eat fast and inattentively, you will make room for negative resonance. So practice slow eating; this way, you will be inviting positive resonance with the archetypes. And, as you'll see with a little practice, we are also the way we breathe. If we breathe superficially, we stay at the surface of life; if we breathe deeply, we go deep in our life. It is that simple. For many people, thinking about their life in these terms can be very revealing.

In conclusion we can say that in order to become healers, we have to apply first of all, the law of resonance to our lives. Also, if we want to help others in our environment (for they are part of our environment too), we have to persuade them to apply the law of resonance in their lives too, because in this way we can see its value, and in this way we can generate positive resonances.

If you have understood this law of resonance, then you will be moved to apply it to yourself. Applying it means a growth of awareness about yourself and an awareness in all the things and people and stimuli in your environment. You will see that this awareness will actually modify the way you look, the way you sit, the way you interact with people, and that all these interactions will also modify constantly your resonance situation inside, the state of your consciousness. And you will discover that attitude, maybe not 100 percent, but a big part of it, is inside. It is mostly the way you are inside. So, if you want to be healthy, happy, and harmonious, try to manifest a healthy and happy inside; try to live more or less in an expanded consciousness. That's a very positive transformation.

When you start to feel unhappy and to display this unhappiness, and you have negativity that shows up in your face, notice the strangeness, and let the negativity go. Don't wait until you are desperate; do you think that kind of desperation ever attracts happiness? Do you think angels (that is how people of the old represented the archetypes; this is codified in our collective unconscious) would ever dare to approach you when you are so contracted? You're too angry for that, you are too strange; they will say (figuratively speaking): "All right, we'll wait here at a safe distance." So develop positivity and be vigilant; remember resonance, remember to apply the principle of resonance in practice.

Patch Adams is a doctor who started some years ago with some of the same observations we are making—now it's an entire trend in medicine, but he started it. Patch Adams started to play with his patients, to make jokes, to do all kinds of funny things to connect with his patients. He was trying to resonate with them, to bring the benefit of his own positive resonance to his clients, instead of adopting the professional coolness that the medical establishment tends to cultivate in medical students, which is insane when you think of it from the perspective of wellness and happiness. Oh, the frustration of doctors who spend all their lives working in laboratories or private practice without having a personal life of resonance and happiness that comes with expansion of consciousness. No wonder when these doctors become older and are in positions of influence, they want to make everybody like them. That is just the way the medical business is run: all objective, right? Mechanical, right? But, this doctor, Patch Adams, broke the pattern and he became very famous because his rate of curing (healing?) was much higher than that of other doctors because he taught his patients how to create a life full of resonance. He didn't explain it in such precise terms as quantum science enables us to explain. He simply said "Smile!" If the patient didn't want to smile, he would keep making jokes, or even play childish pranks, until the patient suddenly would break into a smile, and then just as suddenly the patient's state of consciousness would start to transform.

Of course, due to the predominance of negative emotional brain circuits, the ego/persona is perverse and in that perverse way, it likes the negative resonances. This is a serious problem, and you have to be aware of it. There are many people who are unaware; although they have a choice to change the resonance condition from negative into a positive one, they still do not change it and not because they cannot but because they do not want to. And of course, you will be amazed by how many reasons they consciously choose not to do it. Nobody says, "Actually, I like to suffer." No, they will complain that they are the victims of life, having so many problems: "I have this disease; I don't know what to do; it is my tough luck; it's my bad karma." And then, "What can I do about it if it is my karma?" Victimhood and helplessness run their life—negative resonance. They sound so melodramatic, but in reality, they are just play acting the victim role, because deep inside, if they didn't like the negativity, they would push it away and try to live their lives happily and be healthy.

Here is a quick list of previous and contemporary research about the importance of using sound and music for developing positivity and healing.

USING FREQUENCY AND SOUND FOR HEALING: WHAT THE RESEARCH SHOWS

Sound and music are one of the oldest modalities of treatment. The fact that the body reacts to various frequencies of sound and light is ancient knowledge, and has been used in many traditions, from shamans' drumming to singing music to modern use of light impulse therapy. Today, in labs, scientists are reevaluating sound and light utilization and tapping into the effect of synchrony between the various vibratory frequencies of the lab with those of a human body on the optimal state of health. Using sound and resonance in holistic healing has led to hundreds of products that use modulated waves (radio, acoustics, etc.) of various frequencies, to help regain the state of health—the state of harmonious natural equilibrium of the human being—overcoming physical, emotional, mental, and even spiritual disequilibrium.

The Old Testament starts with: "In the beginning there was the

Word, and the Word was God." In the Indian tradition, the declaration "nada Brahman" reveals the sonar aspect of manifestation of wholeness. In India, there is the tradition of *surat sabd* yoga that teaches people how to listen to inner beautiful sound (*surat* meaning beautiful and *sabd* meaning sound in Hindi).

In India, people have been using sounds in the form of mantra chanting for millennia for the purpose of healing. The mantra ritual resonates with the healing archetype in our collective unconscious.

In the video *Of Sound Mind & Body: Music & Vibrational Healing*, scientist Rupert Sheldrake says that human bodies are "imbricated hierarchies of vibrational frequencies" that are part of a vast and complex vibrational structure. Is he referring to a kind of network of stratified vibrational realities found in the chakras as a basis for a healing system like vibrational medicine? We don't know, but of course, in quantum science we cannot associate the chakras with higher and higher frequencies of vibration as we go up the spine from the root chakra. On the other hand, quantum science does support the idea of vibrational structure in some of our body parts.

Cymatologist Jeff Volk has discussed using cymatics—the study of wave phenomena, especially sound waves and their visual representations—for strengthening the nervous system and the physical body. He mentions such treatments as sonar facial lifting, which harmonizes and strengthens the skin while releasing toxins, and healing the ligaments and joints (as for serious sports injuries). The effectiveness of these uses could be examples of resonance.

In 1950, the English naturopath Dr. Peter Guy Manners correlated the resonating frequencies of healthy tissues and organs (the inner sound that you can become aware of if you practice sabd yoga) and conceived a way to transmit them using sonar ultrasound waves upon the affected tissues and organs. The process he invented is called "sympathetic resonance," and it works the same way as a healing mantra does, as the affected areas are brought back to their original, healthy state that produces the inner sound.

The developing of EEG and EKG measurement techniques increased the possibilities of using sonar audible sounds for healing even the brain, and the work of Robert Monroe consolidated the use of sound frequencies for modulating the brain waves.

Tibetan bowls are used to calm the mind and even induce certain transformed state of consciousness (when the brain vibrates in low frequency theta [3-7 Hz] and delta [1-3 Hz] mode). Studies at the Center for Neuroacoustic Research and the Human Sciences Institute in California have shown that the sound vibrations of dolphins, Tibetan bowls, and even a musical chorus can have healing effect on humans.

Another idea is to discover the chakra resonances and reharmonize vital energies at the chakras. The malfunctioning of a chakra software can lead in time to disease and disequilibrium both at the physical, and also at the mental level.

Meditation researchers and practitioners have noticed healing effects while reciting certain mantras, such as AUM, that would include a state of expansion of consciousness and increased lucidity. The repetitive nature, the rhythm or lyrics of the word repeated, the rituals used, all can have powerful effects upon our bodies and minds. This healing tradition is called mantra yoga.

The late neurologist Oliver Sacks researched the healing power of music and found "profound connection between music and brain" and also that simply chanting can be a medicine as we age. Music affects various parts of the brain. This is why Sacks stated that music is important for us partly due to the way it helps us build memories and learn. He presented the case of a man with Parkinson's disease, who "was able to dance or sing, even though in the absence of music, he was not able to walk or even say a word."

But it's important to remember that we can resonate with music in a negative way too; for example, loud and disturbing music can make some people contract in consciousness and even become physically ill, including vomiting.

A NOTE TO OUR READERS: KEEP A JOURNAL

A journal represents one of the most efficient modalities to mark the important stages of your development in well-being and happiness. It helps you document in written form everything that happens to you from an integrative perspective. It is important to write down the revelations, difficulties, surprises you experience while practicing the methods given in this book. Let yourself be inspired and write what you feel without rational censoring. In this way, you will be able to relax and amplify a certain state of superior receptivity, being more and more in an authentic dialogue with the self of your heart, rather than listening to the chaotic and ever-changing (mostly negative) opinions of the rational mind.

chapter five

WHO IS A HEALER?

There is more to being a healer than being in expanded consciousness: The principle of reflection is the entrance requirement for a true healer; you have to reflect confidence to your client. First of all, to be a healer of others you have to be a self-healer as well, have to know how to heal yourself from negative resonances: You cannot have the tendency to fall into all kind of strange negative resonances and tell a patient, "Be optimistic. Yeah, you are a little bit pessimistic because you are so ... stupid." Because definitely with that attitude you've harmed the guy.

The only true healer in this world is the one who has healed himself: If you cannot heal yourself from negative resonances, if you fall into strange moods and you are still at the mercy of influences regarding your mood swings, you can qualify only as an apprentice healer. If you look upon your body-conglomerate as the source of everything that exists, instead of looking at the state of the body as a consequence of everything that exists, you don't qualify at all. You can be a medical professional approved by your profession, but you are not a healer.

If you don't value two fundamental principles—the principle of resonance and the principle of reflection—and have not applied them successfully to the transformation of your own being, you won't be fully effective as a healer and your attempt to help others will be compromised. Ask yourself: How can you speak about something or apply something that you don't fully know?

There is a story about Mahatma Gandhi that illustrates this point which I (Valentina) heard from a wonderful self-healer. People were going to Gandhi to ask him thousands of favors. It was known that Gandhi's power of persuasion was immense. In one case, a family went to ask Gandhi to persuade their small child not to eat sugar. The child was suffering from diabetes, and because the family didn't give him sweets, he would go out begging on the streets and strangers would give him sweets, thereby aggravating his condition.

Gandhi agreed that it was very good that the family had chosen to ask him to intervene, but told them to return in one month, and then he would talk to the child. The family went back home and then returned in a month as instructed, and since India is a big country and they lived far away, that meant a lot of traveling. When they reached Gandhi again, after standing many hours in a queue, Gandhi took the young boy on his lap and said: "Listen, it is very bad for you to eat sugar. Stop it!" The parents went away satisfied, the boy's reaction was positive, but Gandhi's assistants were confused and furious with him. "That's all?" they said. "For that little advice you made them travel back and forth from their distant village?" Gandhi replied, "Yes, that's all. Now it's only his choice."

"But why didn't you tell him that last month?" Gandhi's assistants persisted. "That was such a simple advice."

"Because last month, I myself was addicted to sugar," Gandhi answered. "I cannot tell a person, 'Don't eat sugar,' and make it count if I myself am a sugar addict. I had to quit sugar first. It took me one month and now I can say it and reflect conviction and inspire confidence."

A person living up to his or her insights is a great soul in this world. In our time, it is people who say, "Walk your talk," because that is the politically correct thing to say in some circles. They do not understand that it is not a question of believing it, but of transformation. Although many psychologists talk about empathy and empathy training, they don't really understand what empathy is or that true empathy demands nonlocality and an ongoing connection of tangled hierarchy. Both walking your talk and having empathy are in fact part of the age-old principle of reflection: You reflect outside yourself what you truly are only to another human being, not to a machine. If you are empathic with the person with whom you are interacting, you are nonlocal—one—with that person, for empathy is quantum in nature. That person may not be as sophisticated as you are, but since you two are one now, she can feel you, and that's the reflection. If she does not feel your conviction, which comes only when you walk your talk, and only when you have transformed, she will not get inspired either. Therefore, if you want to heal somebody, if you want to help somebody to explore the archetype of wholeness, first you have to help yourself with that archetype, heal yourself, and embody wholeness within you.

Of course, you have to remember, this will take time. Rome was not built in a day. It is okay for a healer to be on the path of wholeness and to learn by teaching wholeness to others, healing others along with themselves.

Actually, all the great healers have noticed that in reality every patient they have healed is somehow a part of themselves (that nonlocality again) and therefore with every patient they heal, they go through a process of healing themselves once again. From the healing process, they heal what they still need to heal in order to achieve wholeness.

This is why the real healers can go on healing; they don't need the motivation of name, fame, and money. Today's physicians experience burnout after a decade or so, but real healers never face burnout.

An aside for seekers of spirituality: If a person on the other side of the world is suffering, we also potentially have a problem; if you are correlated with that person, her problem becomes yours. An entire branch of spirituality has developed around this idea. In Tibetan Buddhism, for example, the whole influence of the great cosmic power Tara is based on this concept of the *Kung-yen Vow*: Until the last being in the universe is liberated, my liberation doesn't make sense. I cannot enjoy the total freedom of the spirit if there is still consciousness trapped into any human's illusion of separateness.

To repeat, a healer is, first of all, a self-healer. A healer is healing himself or herself all the time to higher and higher levels of wholeness. And of course, what happens is very interesting: When we are like this, in nonlocal tangled hierarchical quantum empathy, then we are much better prepared to see disease in others, to see what the real problem is, but we have to accept that other people, especially those who are correlated with us in an ongoing way, can see our problems as well. Usually we don't accept this. This is the reason why we don't understand our relationships with other people.

When you have this self-healing walk-your-talk attitude and quantum empathy, you will be amazed how people will just flock to you—and they won't have to say anything; and even if they flood you with a lot of words and information, you'll be able to cut through that directly and see what is the truth.

Sometimes there is nothing true in what clients say. They'll tell you, "You know, I suffer of this and I have this problem, and I suffered when I was little and I have that problem," but actually you can see clearly that no, what they're saying is not true, that it's just an illusion. And, of course, you will have to have a discussion with the client and straighten them out.

Somebody observing that discussion might be surprised by your findings: "How did you know? The person was very honest, the person was crying, the person seemed so very persuasive. How could you know that beyond that there's another problem? How did you point out the problem so very exactly and yet give the client a chance to discover it themselves? How did you do all that?"

Well, it's not such a big deal, it's actually a very simple thing: You know the truth because you know it in yourself, you can see the problem in yourself. Every problem you see in the world around is teaching you about yourself.

There's a story about the Buddha that I (Valentina) heard at a spiritual healing camp I was attending in Europe many years ago. When Buddha went out of his palace and met the fundamental sufferings of life—disease, old age, death—and the way out—renunciation—he didn't say, "Oh, look! This guy is dead, people are dying." No, what he said was, "Look! This guy is dead and I am dying too." And he said: "This guy is suffering; I am suffering too." Later, he sat under the Bodhi tree and became enlightened by taking in these things, healing himself from the fundamental aspects of the human condition that bring us suffering—the things he had never before found inside of himself, but which he found outside the palace where he had lived the very happy life as a prince. With the right attitude, Buddha healed himself, and then he gave humankind a path to heal these fundamental problems with his four Noble Truths. He didn't start to preach, nor did he declare himself as the Buddha before he had succeeded in healing himself of the base-level human condition all the way to reach nonattachment.

A healer does not need to be a Buddha, nor does he need Buddha-level nonattachment, but he or she will be more dedicated, more enthusiastic, and more effective with the acceptance of the healing path to transformation as part of a healer's occupation.

HEALING VS. CURING PAIN: WHAT'S WRONG WITH TODAY'S CULTURE?

It has become part of our medical culture not to look upon the status of health but to focus upon the disease. So let's examine the consequence of this attitude: First, let's consider pain. When nothing is painful, we just live life unconsciously. We never take a look on the status of our health or of our happiness. We never ask ourselves, "Is my consciousness expanded or mostly contracted?" We never check on any of this until something is wrong, and then we check. This is how people use their cars also. They drive their car unmindfully, sometimes even crazily. Then, when something is broken, they think, "Woops, I'd better take it to a mechanic to fix it." The same attitude prevails when we deal with pain by trying to cure it by curing the symptoms.

Our whole life becomes an ongoing battle to remove pain. Well, this is a terribly big mistake from the point of view of consciousness and happiness. Realize this: Pain can be your best friend, because pain is giving you feedback like your best friend. Not everybody has pain, but if pain is the case with you, make that pain your best friend and heed its message. If you did not consciously go through growing pains, you would never have reached maturity. Your consciousness would start to contract (rot?) and it would stink to you and everybody who comes in contact with you. Why else would people avoid you, giving you the feeling that you are unloved? The truth is, you avoid yourself and you can't be at ease with yourself any more. Unawareness does that to you. It is a major contributor to the loneliness epidemic today. Studies after studies show that loneliness is not healthy.

By the time the liver gives any sign of pain, it is already about 80 percent structurally and functionally destroyed Yet, we still don't take care of the liver or try to rebuild it. Instead, we try to fix the pain, and so on the body goes with all the pain we suffer. All of the pain signals given by the body are emergency signals. Pain is an ultimatum we get from nature—so pay attention. Your body is telling you: "Hey, you are going terribly wrong now in your choice of lifestyle and I cannot take it anymore." And on comes pain.

It is like a sign on a highway saying Dead End ("end dead" would perhaps make it clearer); it might become even more annoying when other signs appear: Dead End in 1 km, Dead End in 500 meters, and so on. Saying, "Ah, come on, remove those signs, I want to drive without any limitations" would be ineffective. Of course, that's your choice, but to most people, the choice is clear: You don't wait till the end before you turn around.

Similarly, pain is a signal telling you: "Hey, this is a dead-end where you are going; if you continue, you will end dead." The choice is clear here as well: You should not fight pain. Instead, turn around and change your lifestyle. Find out what is wrong and heal it. It is a fundamental mistake, perpetrated by most people in our current culture when dealing with disease, to look upon disease as the main thing to solve and not focus upon the health as a main thing to keep.

Highway managers know the culture; so today they can repeat a sign; and sooner or later people will notice it. But in the case of health, the managers, the doctors also believe that the disease is it: Just cure it! Often curing it will create other diseases, side effects, but no matter. When you have only a hammer as your tool, you can't do anything but treat everything as nails.

Oh, some physicians do talk about making lifestyle changes, about changing the way you live to heal yourself of chronic disease. But of course in the worldview of material monism, these physicians are coupled with their own solipsistic arrogance and they believe and accordingly treat the clients as mechanical machines. There is no "I" with causal efficacy there that lives; the client's system is all a machine. How can such a client change his lifestyle if there is nobody there, if the client has no casual power?

The attitude we have within our life and towards our life is most of the time an attitude of getting everything we can and paying nothing if it's possible. We want to get pleasure, avoid pain. If pain happens anyway, we want to cure it and move on with further exploration of pleasure—at no cost if possible. This is the attitude of discount hunters, they are constantly looking for discounts on everything they buy, and even form an addiction to these discounts. Well, actually most of the people have this kind of attitude, that's why it is said in every marketing book: "Nothing sells better than discount." Discount is the absolute king of sales on this planet. And this attitude works even with extremely wealthy people. We all want to live cheaply.

Health is no exception. Our attitude that everything had better be cheap—and easy—invades our attitude toward healthcare. For this reason, we only want to feel good without any further investments, without any efforts. The allopathic physician is in cahoots with big pharma offering health cheap and easy, as easy as taking a pill often.

Big pharma has been developed through the perversion of people and culture; it takes advantage of our lack of caring about what is really happening within the human body whenever there is pain. People simply want a pill to solve their problem and big pharma caters to this, making grotesque profit. The pharmaceutical industry thrives but it is the real killer, the reason why we have so many diseases.

We need to realize that in fact we generate our diseases, especially chronic diseases, and perpetuate them. If we change our worldview—and the quantum science for such a change is already here—and if we live with what we have discovered, we can have a happy life on this planet without disease.

The truth is, we have known for millennia how to heal naturally most of the things that go wrong with our health, and this body of knowledge is still growing. We understand the theory of natural healing now. In the old tradition, people did not know much about bacteria, viruses, antibiotics, or physical hygiene (which was not really needed because cities had not yet developed to create so much pollution). And yet, we have a strange situation. The production of medicine is growing almost exponentially. It is a multibillion-dollar industry. The lifespan is longer, with people living to older ages now than at any other time in history. You may wonder how it is possible that we have more medicine and more diseases, statistically speaking, yet we live longer lives. But ask yourself: longer lives to enjoy what? More diseases? After repeated chemotherapy, after ingesting many pain-relief pills and suffering their side effects, after being sent to a nursing home for showing the slightest sign of dementia, what happens to your quality of life?

We are not saying that life at any cost is not worthwhile. Life does have its pleasures, and for many people that compensates adequately for the pain. What we are saying is that you should have the choice, and that there is an alternative. Physicians become real healers when they give their clients a choice in a responsible way, when they themselves have used that choice for self-transformation.

Can we shift the attitude of an entire culture that is reinforced by the media and politics? Only if the professionals wake up to reality. We are not exaggerating; the remedy is simple but people won't see it without the help of you, the healer: Just grasp the quantum perspective of life and health, shift your attitude and learn how to live it. Then teach it to others by healing them. That is the lasting way to heal the culture as well.

LONG ON LIVING, SHORT ON WISDOM

When the average lifespan was only fifty years, people lived until contracting their first serious disease in old age, and that first disease was usually also their last one. You would have a heart attack when you became old, and then you died, and that was that. You'd learn a lesson by watching older people die of disease: Never get a disease! But these days, we have eighty years to "enjoy" lots of pain, disease, tormenting situations of deterioration and dementia after reaching the age of fifty. But of course, doctors and Big Pharma will give you pills that provide temporary respite from your disease. So your disease does not last. You get a little bit cured, and then, once again, you have another bout with disease. More pills. It's a terrible thing that the pharmaceutical industry, the medical practitioners, and ultimately, the materialist worldview are doing to you: They are robbing you of your quality of life for profit.

In antiquity, there was a common phrase, "Memento mori"—"Remember that you are mortal." Caesar Augustus said, "Memento mori" to anyone who came to see him. It was not his way to impose authority; rather, it was his way to make people remember that life is short and you must live wisely, following certain principles and values, because otherwise you'll fall into a miserable state of having no quality of life. In antiquity, life and death went together; people knew that if life happened to you, you could count on death as well. Wise people didn't hang on to life so much, and many lived that life intensely and with quality. They became inspirations and created the values that gave us civilization that we are now destroying with our current attitude.

Nowadays everybody has life insurance. Most people in rich

countries have health insurance. What is health insurance? They should call it "disease insurance" because the insurance companies reimburse you the money you paid if you incur expenses to cure a disease but generally do not keep you in good health. Insurance companies don't reimburse the expenses you incur to maintain good health—education, healing practices, alternative preventive medicines and supplements, positive therapy. They don't give you a discount or even pay you respect: "Congratulations, you're living in good health."

Insurance companies should be honest and call health insurance "disease insurance" because they give you the money when you are ill, not when you are healthy. But how did we develop a culture like that?

You know, a young person starting to pay health insurance besides hospitalization insurance is a person who is perversely thinking, maybe I will get ill, and then I will get my money's worth. Well, congratulations. According to the law of resonance dictated by quantum science of consciousness, you will get ill. Incidentally, health insurers count on young people being healthy. Otherwise, the business will fail. Only a very small percentage of young people who are insured apply for claims. Hence, data shows that young people with insurance are by and large healthy. Chances are, if you are young and have health insurance, you will not get your money's worth.

But if you think, "Why should I pay unnecessary health insurance since I am young and healthy and want to stay healthy? And as soon as I start getting out of health, I will come back to it," then the system will resist and try to impose preconditions.

Some of this is changing in America and elsewhere; Europeans already have government-paid healthcare. But that, too, is fraught with problems because of rapidly rising healthcare costs. In effect, only rich countries can afford healthcare. This is a question of economics.

When life is cheap but we hang on to it no matter what quality it brings, when we are attached to our life at all costs (which health insurance is paying for anyway) and we are desperate to live, even with misery, a funny thing happens: We don't live at all because we are too busy keeping ourselves alive.

The German psychiatrist Alois Alzheimer discovered what we know today as Alzheimer's disease, in 1907. His patient was a forty-three-year-old woman who didn't know where she was and what was going on. Dr. Alzheimer became very interested in her strange status of health and created a daily questionnaire for her. Each day, he asked her the same questions, and he noticed that the answers were getting simpler and simpler until finally there remained only one answer to all of his questions: Augusta, Augusta, Augusta.... Augusta was the patient's name. She couldn't remember anything else except that. In the end, she couldn't even remember her name, and she died.

Many people are reaching old age today. But ask them: "Can you briefly tell me the conclusion of your life?" They are likely to answer with their own names, like Augusta, that first Alzheimer patient.

When we fear living and dying, then we start to fight with the pain, because we want to have an easy life. People think: No matter what, let's have it easy. This is the reason why, most of the time, we go for compromises. All of us are born with the same quantum potentialities, but then we start making choices, and most of the choices we make are according to the prevalent socio-culturally conditioned ideas. Finally, we end up with that attitude of compromising. In reality we know, especially in the beginning, that we are ignoring consciousness and foregoing our infinite potentialities to explore, but after making many compromises, we start to get confused. Then we buy the whole package that the culture offers and accept the human condition; we "enjoy" the cheap and easy life, and then in the end we get disease after disease—and die.

We have in our body a built-in system that is much better than the entire pharmaceutical industry in keeping us healthy. But we don't use it because we are afraid. We shut it off by making compromise after compromise after compromise. And then the things we have there at our disposal, which were super active when we were born, start to become inaccessible. Actually, we do not even call for it: Our fear of living and our fear of dying is shutting off, one by one, all these natural healing mechanisms, and then in the end, we become paralyzed in a crippled soul, a crippled mind, and eventually a crippled body, taking more and more medicine, making more and more compromises. Eventually, in the end, we erase everything as dementia sets in. Why? Because life was not worth living, so it is not worth remembering.

You are a healer when you see all these problems clearly, when you have made an attitudinal shift to the quantum worldview and are living it. Now you can educate and wake up your client before even starting his or her health management. You can say:

"Your attitude is generating all this perpetuation of suffering. What you need to do is to get your life back, start living your life, explore your infinite quantum potentialities. And to get your life back means it comes together with its meaning and purpose served, and you have your terminal disease, you are ready for your death. With this attitudinal shift, you will never fear pain. You will never fear death. You will see both as opportunities. Opportunities for health, opportunities for happiness, even abundance."

In antiquity, people did not look at pain as something which had to be removed. Pain was a phenomenon. They were very curious about it; they did experiments upon themselves. "Hmm, this is pain…interesting." They tried all kind of mechanisms in their body. "If I press here, it is deadly painful; if I press there, it is pleasant." You know, nowadays we only touch the pleasant spots, we never touch the painful spots. We don't usually even recognize that there is a painful spot there at all, and then when we finally do, we just go to the doctor and say, "I have pain. Remove it."

This attitude is generating illness both inside of us and outside. Our society is sick from the same cancers that are making people sick inside. Our culture is a disease of not living enough. Even cancer itself is a disease of not living enough, of not daring enough, of not having the power to embrace all of life, not fully, only a little bit. When you reject life out of fear and lack of love, life turns about to support your cancerous cells more than it supports you. This is how it spreads inside of a person.

If you analyze what people who got healed from cancer did, you'll find that indeed they did many things: some people drank juice, some people did yoga, some started forgiving. There were many methods they used, but all of them developed a certain character trait when they got healed. That all-important character trait is purposiveness: These people have a higher purpose in life, they are committed to higher needs. In the beginning, they didn't have that and they suffered, but they changed and now they have a new lease on their life. You are a healer when you live a life of meaning and purpose and teach your clients the importance of purpose in their life if they want health and happiness.

When you try to help and heal a person, don't even try to prescribe herbs or anything before you have a talk with that person to gauge if they have a vision about their personal life. You need first to understand how much that person really lives his life, how much she is ready to make compromises, whether he has a cheap attitude of only wanting to kill the pain and so on. This is the first obstacle you will face in the process of healing, so work on opening your client for a big attitudinal shift. Only then can you offer her treatments and teach her yoga, meditation, quantum healing—the whole gamut, as needed—and only then will you see her succeed in healing.

Meanwhile, we all—healthy people and sick people, healers and regular people—need to try to change our culture. Healthcare that requires hospitalization has huge costs beyond what an average person can be expected to pay. So, the government has to help. This part of the problem requires political activism to change. But the other part—the attitudinal shift—is our responsibility, both the healers and those being healed.

So, you want to be a healer? Then you have to heal yourself of the wrong machine worldview, heal your own mind, and then walk the talk. Your clients will listen and make the necessary changes—and the culture will change too.

PART TWO

THE QUANTUM SCIENCE of HOLISTIC HEALTH and PREVENTIVE MEDICINE

chapter six

VITAL BODY MEDICINE: GENERAL PRINCIPLES, ACUPUNCTURE, AND HOMEOPATHY

The concept of vital energy was discarded in Western biology and medicine because of the implied dualism and the advent of molecular biology, which made it seem like we could understand everything about the body through the chemistry of DNA, protein, etc. But DNA or protein alone cannot explain healing. As every physician and patient knows, healing not only requires curing physical symptoms but also restoring vitality and vital energy. Vital energy is not the product of body chemistry. Chemistry is local, but the feelings of vital energy, the feeling of being alive, is quite nonlocal. Also, feelings are unreasonable, not computable. But if feelings and vital energy are nonphysical, where do they come from?

A fundamental component of healing is regeneration—even after a severe wound, and the destruction of a massive number of cells, the body has the capacity to regenerate these cells exactly, differentiated as before to perform the particular function as needed. But if you believe this happens because the body has a supply of stem cells, think again. The stem cells are undifferentiated cells, so how do they get differentiated? Regeneration is possible only because our cells' vital software and physiological functions come from nonlocal and nonphysical liturgical fields, and consciousness uses them to differentiate the stem cells as required for cellular regeneration.

Molecules obey physical laws, but they know nothing about the context and functions of living—which includes maintenance and survival, love or jealousy—that occupy us much of the time. The vital body gives us the context of living, which belongs to a separate subtle world that contains the blueprints of vital software that programs organ physiology.

Physical objects obey causal laws and that's all we need to know in order to analyze their behavior; I (Amit) call their behavior law-like. Biological organs not only obey the laws of physics but also perform certain purposive physiological functions: self-reproduction; survival; the maintenance of the integrity of the self, vis-à-vis the environment; love; self-expression; thinking; intuition; and self-knowledge. Some of these functions are easy to recognize as instincts that we share with animals. Others, like thinking, intuition, and self-knowledge, belong only to us humans as a result of further evolution. For example, fear is a feeling that is connected with our survival instinct, but can you imagine a bundle of molecules being afraid? Molecular behavior can be explained completely within physical laws without giving them the attribute of fear. Fear is the vital bodily movement that we feel, and concomitantly, the vital software program for the cells of a physical organ to carry out appropriate physiological functions in response to a fear-producing stimulus.

The behavior of biological systems is interesting because the vital software that programs their physiology is not related to the physical causal laws that govern the movement of their molecular substratum. I call this behavior program-like.

So the vital body is the reservoir of liturgical fields, the blueprints of the epigenetic vital software for the programmed physiological functions. The software programs the turn-on of suitable cellular genes as needed to make the necessary proteins for the organ's function. In this way, the epigenetic software and the organ physiology and hardware perform functions of living—maintenance, reproduction, etc.; and the vital software—conditioned liturgical fields—provide the movement of the energy that we feel as the organ is called in and out of performing a function.

It makes sense. If living forms are run by software programs, then the programs must have started from some blueprints created somewhere by some programmer. Sure, the programs are now built into the hardware as physiology, and the program-like behavior of biological form is automatic. It is easy to forget the origin of the program-like behavior and the programmer. But when the programs of built-in physiology and correlated vital physiology go awry or the hardware is damaged and the vital software cannot connect anymore to the hardware, what then?

The representation-maker, the programmer, is consciousness. Consciousness uses the vital blueprints—the liturgical fields—to make the vital software of organ physiology; the laws of movement of the liturgical fields are codified in the supramental body, body of laws, and archetypes (Figure 8). When consciousness actualizes a physical organ to carry out a physiological function, it also actualizes the conditioned liturgical fields of the vital software, the movement which we feel as the vital energy of a feeling, and of course the archetypal laws governing the whole thing.

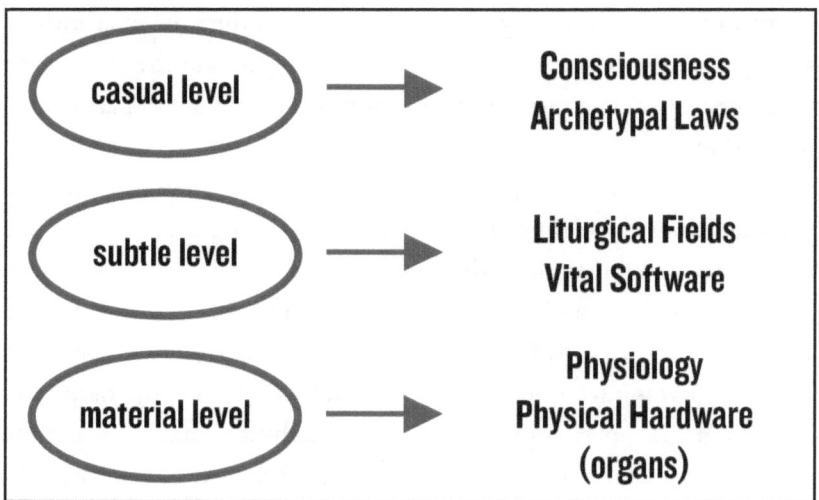

Figure 8. How biological functions come down from heaven (the supramental domain) to earth (the material domain).

Important reminder: The conditioning of vital software covers a spectrum of choices of liturgical fields with varying probabilities. In this way, little changes in the environment can produce a different choice of vital software and a little change in the physiology. This is why, as you experience mood shifts in response to a stimulus, you always find a physiological change as well. Somebody admires your beauty and you blush.

What is *prana*, or *chi*, or vital energy? It is the conditioned quantum movement of the vital body blueprint represented in the V-organ correlated with a physical organ (see Figure 2). When you have the experience of an emotion, there is not only thought but also an extra, subtle, vital movement that consciousness actualizes in your internal awareness: This is manifest prana that is connected to an organ function.

Confusion is created because of the brain's takeover of the functions of the chakra organs for more efficient execution. It seems that the brain is responsible for your emotional response. You need to correct that assumption of conventional science.

Emotions involve internal vital body movements at the chakras in addition to the movements of the mind—thoughts—and the brain's negative emotional circuits. Next time you are angry, and your angry thoughts arise—"I will show him!"—watch out! There is something else, something more subtle, that you also feel internally in the body, that seems to be energy of some sort. That's prana, the vital energy in the appropriate body chakra. The brain circuit is a trigger for this energy, which is in the body.

Is it possible to feel somebody else's feeling? You bet, through quantum nonlocality of the vital body (akin to mental telepathy); we call it empathy. Is it possible for a person of healthy chi to help another balance his or her chi? Yes, again, through quantum nonlocality. This is what Reiki healers do, for example. Their palms are gifted with much vital energy that they transfer to a patient with a sweeping gesture, replacing "bad" chi with "good" chi.

The vital body is indivisible; it has no micro/macro division, no structure. That is why feelings of the vital body are quantum, subtle, experienced internally. However, we acquire vital software through repeated use and resultant conditioning—certain vital movements are conditioned to recur through repeated use, forming a pattern of individual habits. The conditioning covers a spectrum of habits, within the range of all the responses to various environmental stimuli responsible for the conditioned response.

Our physical and vital (and mental and supramental) bodies are separate substance bodies that go on parallelly, with the parallelism maintained by consciousness. But don't picture the substances these bodies are made of as solid or concrete. This is not the quantum way of thinking of substances, not even physical substances. All substances are possibilities—only with collapse as actuality does consciousness give them all the substantiality they have. For the physical, the substantiality is often structural, quite concrete, like our individual physical body. For the vital (and the mental), even the individuality is functional, guaranteeing that they remain subtle all the way, even in manifestation. The substance of vital feeling is vital energy; the substance of mental thought is meaning.

FURTHER EVIDENCE FOR THE QUANTUM NATURE OF THE VITAL BODY

The ancient Chinese researchers noticed that the basic entity that we feel in the vital body, the vital energy that the Chinese call chi, has a complementarity built into it. They named chi's two complementary aspects *yin* and *yang*. You can see quantum insight in the Chinese view. Yin is the transcendent, wavelike character of chi: expansive, nonlocal, creative, "heavenly." In Tai chi, this character shows up when the dancer is still. Yang is the immanent, particle-like character of chi: contracted, localized, conditioned, and "earthly." Yang is experienced when the dancer moves. Both yang and yin aspects are needed to express the full potency of chi, the Tao of chi.

Traditional Chinese Medicine talks about pathways called meridians for the flow of chi from one vital organ to another; the acupuncture points used in Chinese medicine lie along these meridians. These meridians are an integral part of the vital anatomy according to Traditional Chinese Medicine.

If the movement of chi in manifestation is thus localized, at first sight it may seem that the behavior of chi is quite deterministic, not creative. But East Indians also have mapped the manifest movement of chi, which they call prana in pathways they call *nadis*, and these nadis do not exactly coincide with the Chinese meridians. (For a visual comparison, see Figures 9a and 9b, showing two of the most important meridians, or nadis.) This is quite consistent with quantum behavior: The pathways of neither tradition are concrete, but mere guidelines for intuitive exploration.

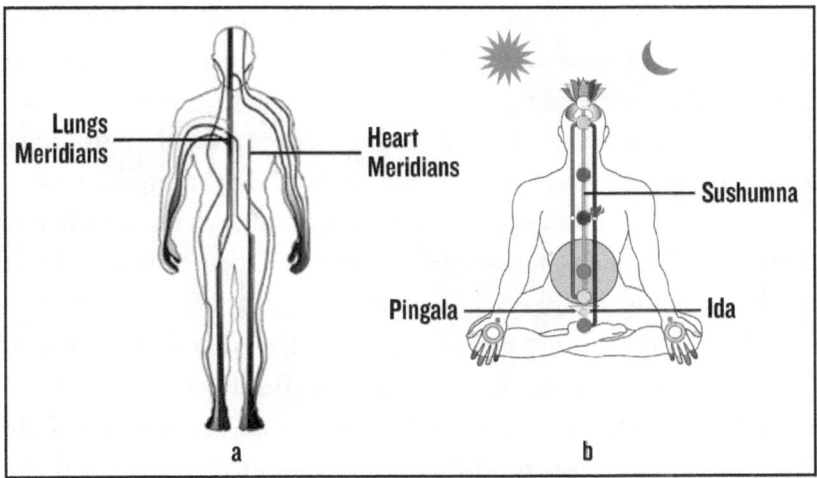

Figure 9. Examples of a) meridians, Traditional Chinese Medicine style, and b) nadis, Ayurveda style.

There may be an uncertainty principle operating between the localization and the direction of movement of chi. Indeed, as mentioned before, the Chinese characterize chi with two complementary aspects, transcendent yin and manifest yang, similar to the complementary characterization of material objects as transcendent wave (of possibility) and manifest particle. When we speak of "balancing the vital energy," in Chinese medicine, it means balancing these yin and yang aspects of vital energy.

ACUPUNCTURE

The best treatment for a physical organ that is affected due to excess or depletion of the movement of chi of its vital software is to direct balancing chi energy to the latter from another vital software belonging to another organ by what seems to be mechanical means—in other words, acupuncture. Traditionally, acupuncture is the most spectacular aspect of Chinese medicine, and currently, the most famous in countries other than China.

I (Valentina) studied acupuncture in Europe with a very charming and dynamic Chinese master. The Latin word *acus* means needle, and *punctura* means puncture; acupuncture is healing by puncturing the body at various points with needles. The place you apply the needle may have no spatial relations to where the disease is. For example, one acupuncturist may apply needles to the big toe to cure a headache, whereas another may do the same using an acupuncture point in the arm. What all this means is that the meridians are not fixed pathways, and using meridians is anything but mechanical, just as quantum physics dictates.

Why do the meridians describe only approximate pathways and why does their use allow so much flexibility and scope for intuition of the healer? Because ultimately, vital energy is quantum in nature and therefore, it is impossible to describe its movement via exact trajectories. This is a dictum of Heisenberg's uncertainty principle. It is also the essential ingredient of the creative process.

Acupuncture was discovered as a byproduct of war. Warriors who were injured by the enemy's arrows made the discovery. They found that although an arrow lodged in the body hurt, it also relieved chronic pains that today we would associate with arthritis, tendinitis, etc. According to legend, when the soldiers' reports reached the Taoist sages, who presumably were experts in Chinese medicine, the latter immediately realized what was happening. In the spirit of true science, they pierced their own bodies with needles and mapped the pathways of chi, the meridians—among them the principal meridians that run from the toes to the head.

An important aspect of the theory is that there are places on the skin where the functioning of these principal channels extends. These are also places where outside influences can affect the organs. The bad news is that external pathogens (for example a cold wind) can affect an internal organ through these areas, too. But we can also apply external energy for healing to an internal organ through the same acupuncture points.

Massage therapy can also be applied through the areas surrounding acupuncture points. In fact, according to some Chinese experts, when acupuncture was first discovered, practitioners used only their fingers to influence the movement of chi. Today, the practice of manipulating chi with fingers is called acupressure.

The meridians are not physical channels at all, nor is anything physical moving through them. Instead, they belong to the vital plane and give us the approximate pathways of movement of vital chi between the vital software of the organs of importance.

Once the vital software that programs the physiological functions of the organ is restored in terms of yin-yang balance and harmony of the relevant chi, the restoration of the organ functions follows quickly.

How acupuncture is actually practiced today supports the quantum view of vital energy. Although traditionalists insist that the meridians are quite fixed as are the acupuncture points, current practitioners agree that rather than being points, the meridians denote areas. Today, acupuncturists do not necessarily use the traditional meridians and acupuncture points. They might ask the patient or even use methods such as muscle testing (a technique of applied kinesiology) to pinpoint where to apply the needles in order to heal the diseased organ.

When I (Amit) underwent acupuncture treatment, Dr. Gopala, my physician, used muscle testing. He would poke places in my left arm and check my right arm muscles for strength or weakness; if the muscles showed strength, he would consider that a hit. That would be the place where he would insert the needles.

How does acupuncture work for relieving headache pain? For a body with healthy organs, the application of the needles to suitable areas stimulates, with creative new infusion, the general level of yang chi (manifest chi) to the body organs, especially to the brain areas that produce endorphins, brain's own opiates. The manifestation of the vitality of chi at the vital level manifest physical brain states with endorphins. Indeed, narcotic antagonist drugs that block endorphins are found to neutralize the healing effect of an acupuncture treatment.

The actual science of acupuncture is designed to heal many ailments, not only headache or pain. In general, acupuncture generates new vital energy possibilities for consciousness to choose from. With intention, a healer can use acupuncture to allow vital energy to manifest at the point of application and to flow from there to the organ at issue to correct its energy imbalance as necessary for healing.

Figure 10 shows one of the principal channels with both the internal and the superficial parts of the pathway. Notice that the superficial branch of the meridians on the arm passes a point above the radial artery of the wrist. This explains how the Chinese medicine practitioner can diagnose disease by reading pulse, which is a highly sophisticated art in Traditional Chinese Medicine, and not coincidentally, also of Indian Ayurveda.

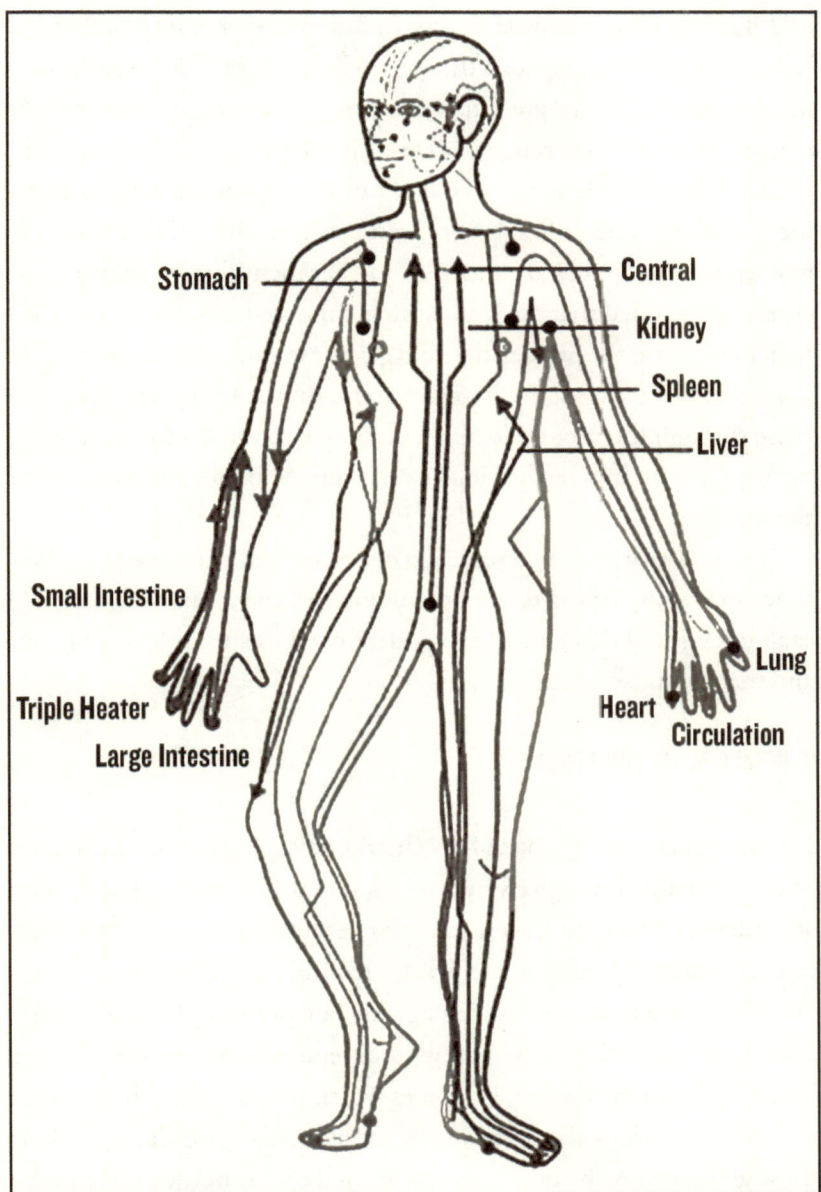

Figure 10. The principal meridians, with both the superficial and interior connections.

Like their Chinese counterparts, traditional Ayurvedic practitioners were also experts in diagnosis through pulse testing (which is really testing the nadis). I (Amit) grew up hearing many fantastic stories about the efficacy of diagnosis through nadi testing. Here is one of those stories.

An Ayurvedic physician was once called by a Muslim king to examine the health of his wife and to suggest a suitable diet. Married Muslim women cannot be seen or touched by other men (family excepted), so custom demanded that the woman sit behind a curtain with a rope tied to her wrist, and the physician would get to examine only this rope (that is, read her nadi through the rope, a chore similar to trying to read her pulse through the rope). However, unknown to the doctor, a trick was being played on him by the king's courtesans, who substituted a cow for the wife.

It is said that the Ayurvedic master examined the rope for a long time, apparently trying to read the pulse, and then said with a sigh, "I can't understand this. But all this patient needs is an ample diet of grass and that will take care of her."

IS HOMEOPATHY FOR REAL?

I (Amit) still remember one of my childhood experiences of the miracle of homeopathy. I was twelve years old, popular, active in sports, good at academics, but I was hugely unhappy because I had an utterly embarrassing thing happening to me: warts growing everywhere on my body. We tried various wart-removing agents, but nothing worked. Finally, somebody suggested homeopathy. I still remember the medicine I got, Thuja 30x—four little white globules which tasted sweet. I had to suck on them until they dissolved in my mouth. After two days of taking these globules, one by one the warts just fell off my body. I was cured. I was so relieved. It was like a miracle.

But at the time I didn't appreciate the entirety of the miracle that homeopathy really is. I did not know that calculations can easily prove that on the average it was unlikely that there was any medicinal substance at all in the dilution of Thuja that I took—at least not in the conventional sense of what we mean by medicine. According to the conventional way of thinking, four little sugar pills cured my disease. Nowadays, a "sugar pill cure" being administered as medicine, so that the patient thinks he is getting something "good" from a qualified healer, is called a placebo cure. Most allopaths, when they hear a story like mine, dismiss homeopathy, saying the pills were just a placebo. What complicates the issue is that many diseases like warts have actually been known to be cured by placebo.

Of course, the placebo also seems to be a miracle cure. To see how the placebo works, think of a disease that occurs when the immune system response is not working properly. A good example is arthritis. Placebo works by triggering the body's defense mechanism to work properly through situational creativity by boosting our healing intention once again.

Is homeopathy a placebo? Many studies have been done and the outcome is still controversial, although I have read that a few studies have been definitive. So let's ask the question in another way? Does homeopathy work? Can it actually work in the face of the allopath's correct criticism that with homeopathy, not even one molecule of the medicinal substance is being administered? And if it works anyway, how does it work? I developed the theory behind homeopathy in *The Quantum Doctor*. Here it is in synopsis.

Two fundamental axioms of homeopathy were discovered by its founder, Samuel Hahnemann. The first axiom is, simply, like cures like. If a certain medicinal substance produces a certain confluence of symptoms in a healthy body, then that substance will act as a cure to a diseased person with the same symptoms.

Even today, homeopathic researchers do their "provings" more or less the way Hahnemann did it in 1796. He took poisonous substances that he had some reason to believe were also medicinal and administered each one in miniscule doses to healthy subjects who noted down all their developing symptoms, which he then matched with the symptoms of known diseases. These provings are still being done today. They then become part of a Materia Medica, which physicians can consult to find the like-cures-like medicines for diseases through similarity of symptoms.

I (Valentina) use homeopathy only rarely but always with success—mostly when a patient's situation is more difficult, or in certain stages of the disease, and a new approach is necessary. For example, I have used homeopathy for treatment of Lyme disease, fibromas, and even stroke. I use homeopathy because it gives me access to an entire new class of poisonous herbs which cannot be used in Ayurveda.

How does homeopathy manage to use poisonous herbs? This is where the second axiom of homeopathy comes in: "Less is more." This is the axiom that aggravates the materialist allopath the most. The more you dilute the medicinal substance in an 87 percent mixture of alcohol in water (using a certain procedure, see below), the more potent the effect is. And the dilutions that homeopaths routinely prescribe for their patients are ridiculous, materially speaking.

Consider this: One part of a medicinal substance is diluted with roughly nine parts of the alcohol-water mixture. This mixture is thoroughly shaken ("succussed," to use the technical term) about forty times; after this, nine parts are discarded, and the remaining one part is diluted once again with the water-alcohol mixture. This mixture is succussed once again, and the process of dilution and succussion may be continued indefinitely producing medicine of increasing potency denoted as 1x, 3x, 6x, 30x, 100x, and so forth.

Allopathic physicians ridicule homeopathy because after a certain dilution it is mathematically extremely unlikely that even one material molecule of the "medicine" will be present.

Let's get a little technical to drive in the allopath's seemingly valid point. Avogadro's Law of Chemistry says that a "mole" (which stands for the equivalent of the molecular weight of a substance in grams) of any substance contains of the order of 10^{24} molecules of the substance. So, after a homeopathic dilution of 24x of a mole of a medicinal substance (which chemically means a dilution by a factor of 10^{24}), it is not likely that there will be a single molecule of the medicinal substance present.

But both axioms make sense from a vital-energy point of view. From the vital perspective, the immune system consists of the physical hardware—vital software for defending the body against external or internal antigens. A disease means that this physical-vital combination, in its current form, is not working properly. It makes sense that this malfunction may be due to the malfunction of the vital software. If the software is missing a few elements, we have to infuse these elements to fix the vital software in the system to effect a cure. The herbs provide the missing elements of vital software.

Like cures like. If the medicinal substance—a live herb—is poisonous, the herbal software will suppress that part of the software from the working software of a healthy person; hence the symptoms. The symptoms are the signature of what is missing. In this way, if a diseased person has the same symptoms, we conclude the person is missing the software in that poisonous herb. Now, do you see? Homeopathy extracts the vital part from the physical this way. It serves the patient just the vital missing software without the poison, which is contained in the molecules. This is the mystery of like cures like.

And now, the principle "less is more" also makes sense—it is the way to isolate the vital from the physical part of the herb. The medicinal substances are often toxic, though not poisonous, at the physical level. If the cure is in the vital plane, the physical is really irrelevant, and what is the wisdom of administering unnecessary toxic stuff to the organism only to produce unwanted side effects? It makes sense to dilute the medicine and eliminate the medicine's physical body while the vital remains intact.

As mentioned, homeopaths use a very elaborate procedure of shaking the mixture before making further dilutions. Even that now becomes plausible. This shaking procedure makes sure that the vital energy, correlated before with the physical part of the medicine alone, now becomes correlated with the water of the alcohol-water mixture.

(How? Through the conscious intention of the preparer, all the succussion movements are helping to maintain that intention.)

Can water make memory-representations of vital energy like a film capturing your picture? Yes, it can. The phenomenon of dowsing proves that. Can our intention transfer vital energy? The great Stanford researcher William Tiller, who studied how intention can transfer vital energy, demonstrated that by direct experimentation.

THE IMPORTANCE OF HERRING'S LAW

There is another homeopathic doctrine of great preventive wisdom: Herring's Law. Without going into details, the import of this law lies in this fact: The physical symptoms of a disease are preceded by the symptoms of vital malfunction, mental malfunction, archetypal malfunction, and eventually spiritual malfunction in that order.

According to quantum science, most breast cancer is due to the vital energy block of love energy at the heart chakra. Most often such vital energy blocks are caused by a mental block giving incorrect mental meaning to a physical-vital event. For instance, a loved one dies and the patient grieves so much as to not accept love energy anymore from anybody. Now apply Herring's Law. Long before the physical symptoms of breast cancer—a lump in the woman's breast—there were spiritual, archetypal, mental, and vital symptoms. So, a woman's cancerous lump is preceded by 1) spiritual disconnect, a general lack of expansion of consciousness in everyday life, which is the first warning sign; and 2) difficulties or disinterest in maintaining intimate love relationships, and not necessarily sexual ones, because the person has lost interest in the archetype of love, specifically; 3) a decision to withdraw love and symptoms of withdrawal from the world—low indifference; 4) low indifference produces a vital energy block at the heart for which the symptoms are very clear: excessive grieving, stubborn lack of forgiveness, etc.; 5) and then only then, physical symptoms.

Look at the import of this in terms of predictive power. Today, 85 percent of people are worldview-confused, causing a general spiritual disconnect. We can immediately predict that the overwhelming majority of these people will end up with some sort of chronic disease. Some of these people who cannot hold a relationship additionally will develop depression. A substantial portion of these people may specifically block the archetype of love; they will be prone to both navel chakra and heart chakra disease (see Chapter 9 for details). If it is only self-love that they block, they may contract chronic diseases of the navel chakra, such as Type II diabetes, in their old age. Finally, those who specifically block other love at the heart may end up with cancer.

USE OF HOMEOPATHY IN THE AFTERMATH OF BACTERIAL OR VIRAL INFECTION AND ALLOPATHIC CURE

By the same token, Herring's Law implies that healing must take place in the reverse order opposite to the progression of disease. So, after an allopathic cure of symptoms, one has to heal the vital body, then the mental body, and so forth.

For prevention, you develop sensitivity and try to catch the symptoms as early in their development as you can and make appropriate lifestyle changes and engage practices.

Under the monopoly of allopathy, a crucial neglect is happening with healthcare: Little to no attention is given to the patient during the recovery period, and patients are left on their own with little guidance about the importance of rest and diet, maybe not even the suggestion of a follow-up doctor's visit. This is a big mistake. A patient must consult with alternative medicine physicians at this stage and receive suitable treatments to heal her other bodies. Only then can healing be holistic and complete.

However, currently there seems to be no consensus among the two most popular alternative systems of vital body medicine—Traditional Chinese Medicine and Ayurveda. One of this book's major accomplishments is the integration of these two systems in a way that also includes Taoist medicine and chakra medicine, which is the subject of the next three chapters.

chapter seven

COMPARATIVE MEDICINE: INTEGRATING AYURVEDA AND TRADITIONAL CHINESE MEDICINE

If you ask an allopathic physician the question, "What's my body type?" he or she will say, "Well, that depends on your genes, doesn't it?" But does it? If you point out that genes are more or less just the instructions to make proteins, not for morphogenesis nor for producing purposive functional physiology for the organs, the allopathic doctor will say in exasperation, "If genes cannot explain it, then there is no such thing as body type. And even if there were, it would not be important. Your disease does not care about how your personal body is constituted unless you have a genetic defect. The treatment does not depend on your so-called body type either."

But human beings, even single-cell creatures, are heterogeneous, the vital software and how effectively it is used does vary from person to person. In medicinal systems that include the vital body—the morphogenetic/liturgical fields that contribute to form-making as well as give purposive function to form—body types make perfect sense. In this way, both Indian Ayurvedic medicine and Traditional Chinese Medicine have very important things to say about body types—the classification of our natural constitutions. They both give guidance about how to take care of your body depending on your body types—for each body type, certain tendencies for diseases develop and the prevention and treatment depends on the body type. Unlike allopathy, vital body medicine is individualized, and this is one of its greatest strengths.

Unfortunately, when you take a look at both schools, the Indian and the Chinese, you may be disappointed at first. The two systems don't seem to agree with the assessments of heterogeneity with one another. Shouldn't science be monolithic?

It is very important to note that since the vital body is subtle, vital body medicine also has to be subtle. We can, generally speaking, only have internal subjective experiences of the subtle. Thus we cannot, in general, expect to have a strongly objective, single-observer independent science for the vital body. At the same time, science requires at least weak objectivity or observer invariance; the conclusions drawn must be independent of a particular observer. The Chinese and the Indian systems have enough points of similarity to satisfy the criterion of weak objectivity of vital body medicine. Once cultural conditioning is taken into consideration, the two systems can be seen to complement, not contradict each other in this way, opening up the possibility of an integrated vital medicinal system.

BODY TYPES IN TRADITIONAL CHINESE MEDICINE

The underlying philosophy of Traditional Chinese Medicine is Taoism with an emphasis on the two-fold complementarity of yin and yang, creative potentiality, and conditioned (within a flexible range) actuality—the software. So the Chinese characterization of body types is twofold: The yang type applies to those who have the tendency to maintain the existing yang, the existing software of the vital stasis and movements within the available flexibility, the existing yin; and the yin type applies to those with the tendency to explore new potentialities, or new yin.

The two-fold distinction of conditioned yang-creative yin at the vital level is quite effective to differentiate body types: moist-dry, heavy-light, slow-rapid, passive-aggressive, still-active, creative/stable, inward/introvert-outward/extrovert, etc.

Most medicinal systems—ancient Greek medicine, Traditional Chinese Medicine, modern homeopathy, and allopathy—assume that human physiology is given to us as a permanent fixture which never changes. In that case, the two-fold classification would have been enough for maintaining health if we take the given human condition as our lot. In this respect, we would be no different than other mammals.

AYURVEDA AND A BETTER ASSESSMENT OF HUMAN HETEROGENEITY: DOSHA IMBALANCES

Ayurveda is a science of health and healing developed in India, where it has been in use for millennia. Thanks to its widespread use today in both India and abroad, as well as its brilliant expositors, such as Deepak Chopra and David Frawley, Ayurvedic concepts such as the doshas have become commonplace in America in the 1990s. I (Amit) remember I was at a party during that period and a complete stranger, a woman, asked me out of the blue, "So what's your body type? Are you a Vata, a Pitta, or a Kapha?" The implication was clear to me. It was the current icebreaker with which to begin a conversation. Before this person would start a conversation with a stranger, she needed to know the person's Ayurvedic typology. In the 1970s, the icebreaker used to be astrology: "Are you a Sagittarius?" In 2020, it was, "What do you think of COVID?"

The fundamental assumption of Ayurveda is that one is born with a given body type—a particular "base level" imbalance (called *prakriti* in Sanskrit) of the three characteristics or qualities (called *gunas* in Sanskrit) that govern our creativity in the vital arena—*ojas*, *vayu*, and *tejas* and their corruptions, the doshas—kapha, vata, and pitta—respectively. These corruptions at the vital level produce manifest defects in the physical level—the physiology—which can lead to disease.

The fact that many children suffer from chronic conditions of illness support the view that there may be innate imbalances of the vital qualities of the tejas, vayu, and ojas producing dosha imbalances that we are born with.

The generic name "dosha" has been used both to denote the qualities as well as their malfunction by some authors, and this creates confusion. Etymologically, dosha means defect, a corruption in the application of the guna attribute. The contingencies of life, lifestyle, and response to environmental stimuli, etc., take a person to the corruption of the attributes during developmental years, producing further imbalance in prakriti. The generic name for the imbalance is *Vikriti* in Sanskrit. It is the imbalance that causes disease. So, again, like Traditional Chinese Medicine, isn't the vayu-ojas balance between creativity and conditioning enough to maintain health, to maintain the physiology we are born with? What is the role of pitta? This, as you will see, is a crucial question, which opens up a new vista for Ayurveda.

A BRIEF HISTORY OF THE TRI-DOSHA THEORY

As with Greek medicine, the early ideas of Ayurveda were probably the result of empirical observation of three body humors (kapha literally translates as phlegm in our respiratory system; vata as intestinal gas; and pitta as acidity in the stomach) and associating them with a physical defect that comes from the blockage or corruption of a vital quality, vital inertia, or ojas; vayu, or the vital quality of situation creativity; and tejas, or the ability of fundamental vital creativity.

> **Kapha:** Maintaining the same old software activities is ritualistic, producing vital lethargy; vital movements lack zing and physical wastes don't get cleared up. The result is phlegm in the respiratory system or cholesterol in the circulatory system. The blockage is called the vital dosha of kapha.
>
> **Vata:** The humor of intestinal gas (vata) was theorized as the product of

the blockage of the vital guna of Vayu that produces the vital dosha of Vata. Excess vata prevents the maintenance of balance between creativity and conditioning required for good organ health.

Pitta: The humor of stomach acidity (pitta) is due to the blockage of the vital guna of tejas; the corresponding vital dosha is called pitta.

The original Ayurvedic researchers were also aware that vata predominates in the lower third of the body below the navel; pitta is predominant in the middle third covering the stomach and the heart; and kapha is predominant in the upper third—the lung, the throat, and the head.

The development of Ayurveda goes back to the Vedic times and it was influenced by the five elements theory of reality then prevalent in India. These five elements corresponded to the five experiences: sensing (physical), feeling (vital), thinking (mental), intuiting (archetypal), and expansion of consciousness (spiritual).

Unfortunately and fortuitously, it just so happens that matter also exists in five states: solid (earth), liquid (water), gas (air), plasma (fire), and vacuum (absence of matter or ether). The vital researchers noted that phlegm was semi-solid—a mixture of the elements of earth (solid) and water (liquid); in this way, the kapha dosha was associated with those two elements—earth and water. Similarly, pitta was associated with liquid and gas; and vata with gas and emptiness or ether. These matter associations played a major role in later development of Ayurveda.

Likewise, Traditional Chinese Medicine developed on the basis of the five-elements theory of the vital—the idea that vital stuff exists in similar five states of matter: earth, water, fire, wood, and metal.

The Chinese used the yin-yang to classify organs, whether an organ is dominated by yang (inertia), or yin (creativity). They used the five-element theory to help figure out how the organs influence one another at the vital level. (This is discussed in detail in *The Quantum Doctor* and will not be repeated here.)

The Ayurvedic theoreticians additionally made the observation that the body is made of seven components (Sanskrit *dhatus*) of *asthi* (empty tubes, site of vacuum or ether or air); rasa (juice); *rakta* (blood), *shukra* (semen); *mamsa* (muscle); *meda* (fat); and *majja* (nerve tissue). The following associations suggest themselves if you use the five-element theory to make the associations as these theoreticians did:

Asthi, majja – vayu, vata
Rasa, rakta – tejas, pitta
Mamsa, meda, majja, rakta, shukra – ojas, kapha

Asthi is usually translated as bone, which causes confusion. However, bone has a lot of empty space in it as do the pipes that carry our solid waste—the colon and the rectum—when you consider that in principle the colon and rectum can be empty and are empty some of the time. And of course, the nerves also have a lot of empty space, and thus are associated with vata.

Rakta (blood) carries oxygen; in this capacity, the argument went, it falls in the category of pitta. However, it also carries the nutrients and is carried by the arteries and veins—and therefore made of solids; in this way, rakta qualifies as both pitta and kapha. Semen is liquid—it has the sperm cells, the basic stuff of the biological hardware, and thus is associated with ojas and kapha. By the way, sperm is called *oujas*—a Sanskrit word that is derived from ojas.

The rest—mamsa, meda, majja—are associated with ojas and kapha as well.

Rasa, translated as juice, was originally associated only with intestinal digestive juices. More recently, however, Ayurvedic researchers have correctly included the immune system juice of lymph in this category.

So the ancients interpreted kapha as a defect in the exercise of the quality of stasis, vata as the defect in the motif for creative movement involving air and vacuum, and pitta as defect in the creative movement of rasa.

Finally, we are getting a hint. Both of the rasas involve the function of two sets of important organs; the first set—digestive organs—belong to the navel chakra. The other, the immune system (in the form of the thymus gland), belongs to the heart chakra.

For further reading of the notions of classical Ayurveda, read the book *Tridosha Theory* by V. V. Subrahmanya Sastri; however, be wary: Don't buy into all of Sastri's ideas because only some of them are compatible with science.

THE QUANTUM APPROACH TO UNDERSTANDING THE VITAL GUNAS AND DOSHAS

This is a problem tackled already to some extent in *The Quantum Doctor*. Neither Traditional Chinese Medicine nor Ayurveda use concepts such as creativity and conditioning. The use of quantum concepts is telling us that vata inhibits creative movement and kapha compromises the stasis of conditioning; in this way, the fundamental ingredient of the creative process we call *do-be-do-be-do*, a balanced tandem application of imaginative vital movements and relaxed stasis, no longer operates properly. For health, we need to balance vayu and ojas.

But then we are back to square one: Isn't a vata-kapha imbalance enough of a basis for discussing all the vital software doshas of human physiology that cause disease? What is the role of tejas? How does pitta arise?

Conventional Ayurvedic wisdom tries to differentiate between ordinary creativity involved in regulating changes in movement in response to environment stimuli and the creativity involved in the conversion of food into body cells. But that is not the point. In both cases, it is the movement of the existing software that has to be guided creatively using its flexibility, and vayu does both.

But first, let's address this question: What is the nature of the software? Is it all universal and fixed? Of course not. There has to be a personal component to the software; people have different imbalances of the creative qualities and different doshas. Nature gives hardware, physiology, and the universal vital software. Nurture gives the personal vital software during development, providing the flexibility we need for situational changes in the environment. Indian philosophy and much recent evidence suggest another source of personal software: reincarnation.

Reincarnation is part and parcel of all Eastern systems of thought, and Ayurveda is no exception. And the idea of reincarnation is scientific: The demonstration of the existence of reincarnation actually proves the existence of the subtle bodies—vital, mental, and supramental—because the modification of the expression of the laws of functioning of these bodies that we live in is what is reincarnated. These modifications, called karma, can theoretically be explained, giving further credence to the idea of reincarnation. Read Amit's book, *Physics of the Soul*, for details.

So, the reincarnational inheritance—the prakriti we are born with—is vital karma; but this is not all of it, there is also the contribution of nurture. Let's spell out the role of nurture. In our formative years, when the body's structure is being built, ojas dominates. Ojas is inertia; it leaves the universal software and prakriti in operation alone. In the middle portion of development, starting roughly at age six, tejas—the ability to engage fundamental creativity—begins to appear. Major individualized form and software-making happens between age six and adulthood. In the late portion of development, when we become adult, vayu dominates—only situational creativity is used in the main to make further changes. As development is over, roughly around age twenty-five, we have a new prakriti—a new balance of the vital gunas and doshas. This is the one that traditional Ayurveda says, if you preserve, you will have good health.

This is all standard Ayurvedic lore dressed in quantum lingo. And still there is no real explanation of the role of tejas and pitta. What does tejas do that vayu cannot do? In other words, using quantum language, what is the role of fundamental creativity in shaping organ function?

Since disease happens more frequently when we are middle-aged and beyond, clearly most disease must be due to vata corruption or aggravation in the dhatu components that house vata: the colon, the nerves, and the bone joints. The next most prevalent disease is due to pitta corruption involving the digestive organs and immune system malfunctions. Disease caused by kapha corruption is the least common, but among them is obesity, which can be pathological. Diseases due to congestion are due to too much kapha and no vayu to clean up because of vayu corruption resulting in vata aggravation.

Our common, modern go-go-go lifestyle aggravates vata and pitta, says traditional Ayurveda. So, on the face of it, Ayurveda gives us a simple message: Watch out for aggravated vata and pitta and you will be healthy.

I (Valentina) studied and practiced Ayurveda and Panchakarma in India at the Dayanand Ayurvedic Hospital and University of Jalandhar with a real Ayurvedic doctor, Sanjeev Sood. I say "real" because, unfortunately, nowadays we find the same materialistic approach toward Ayurveda that we find in allopathy: production in bulk. Instead, we need to go in a different direction. Quantum science is taking us to properly grasping the nature of Ayurvedic healing, bringing forth freshness and depth to this ancient science. We are cowriting this book while we develop a course on integrative medicine for our Ph.D. students, and it feels as if all the dots are falling in the right place.

I learned that the practice of Ayurveda needs to be more subtle than this indicates. Even modern allopathic medicine has begun to emphasize lifestyle (the social theory of disease). For example, heart disease is associated with so-called type-A personality and lifestyle (hyperactive, overanxious, do-do-do) even by allopathic physicians. However, the personality refers to the defect in emotional response caused by how we use the mind in response to stimuli that activate the negative emotional brain circuits. Ayurveda, on the other hand, is talking mainly from the vital body side of things.

The approach of Ayurveda takes account of the fact that not everybody with a type-A personality gets heart disease. Ayurveda attempts to bring the patient back to its base-level dosha distribution, to his or her prakriti at the end of body development. If the base level is already type-A, Ayurveda does not bother to correct it. It is not going to be any problem. It is this personalized nature of Ayurveda that makes Ayurveda useful in treating disease, but not necessarily chronic disease. In that department, Ayurveda can do better with proper understanding of how tejas and pitta work.

What is the scientific basis of this idea of tejas guna and pitta dosha, or is there any? Modern Ayurvedic practitioners avoid this question, but we give a scientific explanation of it in this book.

THE QUANTUM SCIENCE OF AYURVEDA

Consciousness collapses vital feelings along with the correlated physical organ for its experiences of living. We have to remember that our physical bodies are in constant flux; our cells and organs are being constantly renewed with the help of the food molecules that we eat. We also have to remember that the quantum possibilities of the vital body consist of a possibility spectrum (with a corresponding probability distribution determined by the quantum dynamics of the situation) of the conditioned morphogenetic/liturgical fields, the blueprints of the vital body software. The dynamical laws of the vital body and organ functions, the contexts of movement of the organ software, are contained in the supramental.

As mentioned earlier, we are all born with a universal software plus some additional personal software from our reincarnational heritage. On our way to adulthood, we make additional software using vital qualities or attributes that we call the three vital gunas:

- Ojas is inertia; no new form or software is added.
- Vayu consists of situational creativity; when the situation changes because of environmental factors, with vayu we can choose a

combination of the available components of the software to find an answer to the problem.
- Tejas, in quantum thinking, consists of the use of fundamental creativity of the vital movements. What does it do? Brings in brand new software for organ function, what else? But what does it mean?

For most of body's functions, for the functions of the dhatus, we don't need new functions. The existing functions are adequate; the challenge of health is to keep the function going. For that we maintain yin-yang balance, a balance of conditioning and creativity, vayu, and ojas.

In other words, kapha and vata are in exact correspondence of the Chinese characterization. Kapha is the tendency for too much inertia; vital activity is there, too much yang, but it is all ritualized, no zing in it, no new potentiality is being actualized, no dynamism. With vayu, we bring dynamism, new yin. Now a balance can be reached. However, again, if there is too much vayu, not enough ojas, then there will be too much creative yin, with not much of it actualized into new conditioned yang, so once again an imbalance of vata and kapha, respectively, results.

To understand the need of tejas and to explain the existence of pitta people, we need a new perspective other than Traditional Chinese Medicine and classical Ayurveda. Tejas and pitta come into play in the navel and the heart chakra organs. Let's look at the theory of the chakras for more clues.

CHAKRA DYNAMIC AT THE NAVEL AND THE HEART

Our feelings are associated with the chakras. At the root chakra, we feel fear or security. The brain take-over gives us the responses of flight or fight corresponding to how we feel.

For the navel, in response to the feeling of hunger, the brain take-over translates into another F-response—feeding. Unbalanced responses generate various feelings connected with negative emotion—anger, greed, pride, and narcissism.

As they grow up, kids have to deal with their physical differences as they learn to be autonomous and interact with other kids. The ojas/kapha dominated kids will be stalky and robust. Reincarnational prakriti will be different from kid to kid, some kids will be tejas/pitta dominated, and some will be vayu/vata dominated.

Watch the bully phenomenon, which is a major challenge of growing up. Bullies pick on some kids, but not others. How do they choose? They pick the ones with the normal navel chakra feelings—insecurity and pride.

Bullies seldom pick on the kids that are confident and have feelings of self-worth. Where does that feeling come from? Chakra psychology tells us the story. These kids have transformed and awakened their navel chakra to a higher functional level that gives them self-worth while they were struggling with autonomy in their childhood.

We submit that this higher functional level is a fundamental change in the functional software of one or more organs of the chakra. And this is due to the fundamental creativity of tejas, a new supramental function has been actualized.

The awakening of the feeling of self-worth signifies quantum self-experience; an explicit self-identity has come about at the chakra. Before this awakening, there was no vital autonomy and the chakra was governed by the brain's self. Now the self at the chakra can be directly experienced in a pure feeling of self-worth.

The study of pitta-dominated adults show that pitta people reach their "high" but then come down, and then they get bogged down with the usual feelings once again. Why? The answer is that the software is there, but it's a choice to use it. Tejas people use it only occasionally. When they come down, if tejas is balanced with ojas and vayu, no problem. Otherwise, the imbalances of the latter will mess things up as usual and tejas will be needed. The pitta dosha prevents that.

Later, at puberty, the challenge of sexuality requires similarly the invocation of tejas to create new form/software at the heart chakra. Boys and girls are naturally attracted to one another and will engage in sex. Occasionally though, a phenomenon called romantic love shows up: The couple involved has their thymus gland (part of the immune system that discriminates between me and not-me) suspended momentarily and the heart wakes up to a new coherent quantum functioning that the couple experiences as an expansion of consciousness to include the other involving the feeling of caring. As people develop the software of loving, the immune system gets frequent rest and begins to function at a healthier level as well—if vayu and ojas are balanced as well at this higher level. These are the people of tejas. People who use the love software only occasionally, and their balance of vayu and ojas is unstable, they suffer from pitta dosha.

In this way, all heart chakra and navel chakra organ disease can be said to be due to pitta aggravation, corruption of tejas.

Note also that the awakening of romance in the heart is a quantum self-experience and signifies the awakening of an autonomous self at the heart chakra (see also Chapter 11).

Exploration of fundamental creativity hugely enlarges the existing repertoire for software or yin—vital potentiality. When adulthood is reached, a person can live counting solely on vayu—the ability for situational creativity of the vital—to counter the ill effects of kapha. But only if a healthy lifestyle is maintained.

The doshas—physical body defects in organ functioning—can happen during this developmental scenario due to situational change of environment due to travel or seasonal change which may bring about minor disease, or fundamental change in severe diseases caused by accidents, bacteria, and viruses, and stressful life style.

After recovery from a minor disease such as a common cold, general weakness of vitality prevails, which calls for lot of new yin to be actualized: creativity. If kapha dominates a child, such will not be the case.

And vital weakness may become a permanent fixture of the child producing congestion in movement of breath—phlegm in the respiratory channel.

If vata is the dominating aspect, then during the recovery from an ordinary disease, too much yin is there without being actualized, causing, again, an imbalance. This is responsible for the obstruction to the movement of stool, feculence—a tendency for passing intestinal gas and other elimination system problems such as constipation—physical dosha of vata.

Finally, consider the recovery from a severe disease. One fallout is lack of appetite due to lack of tejas. It requires a lot of tasty spicy food to re-activate tejas. But if tejas is corrupted and the person suffers from pitta, the excess spicy food tends to produce excess acidity.

You can see how the names of the doshas came about from the nature of how these physical doshas affect our breathing and food habits required for the maintenance of the body.

To summarize: The particular combination of dosha imbalances that we develop as we grow up, our physical prakriti or body type, is a homeostatic combination of what we are born with and what our early development to adulthood, when the physical body stops growing, contributes. In traditional Ayurveda, our physical body functions optimally when we remain at this homeostasis. If, however, our vital tendencies to produce further imbalances are not corrected and are allowed to continue unabated, deviations from this homeostasis take place and disease at the physical level is due to this movement away from the homeostasis.

In this way, Ayurvedic healing can take two tracks. First, the obvious one: Correct the physical problems arising from the dosha imbalance beyond dosha prakriti at the beginning of adulthood at the physical level itself. Some of the Ayurvedic treatments are designed with this in mind; panchakarma, a cleansing of the body, for example. But this healing is only temporary and has to be done regularly.

The other track is to correct the vital body imbalance-producing tendencies, for which correction alone can lead to permanent remedy. This other track can be practiced in two ways—passive and active. The passive path is accomplished through food and herbal medicine; Ayurvedic physicians administer food and herbs of specific software patterns of prana to compensate what is missing. The active path is to transform the movements of prana at the vital body level directly. Breathing practices called pranayama, in which one watches the movements of breath along with the associated vital prana movements along the meridians that connect the different vital organs, and Tai chi, alternative movement (of mainly hands and arms) and stillness at the physical level, are prime examples of the active path. Reiki masters can also move energy between the chakras using the meridians to heal chakra imbalance by passing their energized palms over a patient's body. The dynamics of vital interaction produce new possibilities giving consciousness a better chance to choose the new healing software.

DISEASE AND HEALING IN TRADITIONAL CHINESE MEDICINE AND AYURVEDA: HERBAL MEDICINE

Generally speaking, we find that both traditional Indian and Chinese systems use general principles about the vital liturgical fields to:

a. define health which is balance and harmony;
b. define disease as the absence of balance and harmony; and
c. derive relationships between the systems of the physical-vital body, which then can be used to develop cures.

Disease that is other than chronic in these medicine systems means imbalances in creative yin and conditioned yang; Ayurveda would say that the former is due to vata and the latter is due to a kapha dosha.

The remedy, first of all, is preventive: Maintain the yin-yang balance in Traditional Chinese Medicine and prakriti in Ayurveda. If this fails anyway, neither of these systems are of much use except to produce some relief. In Quantum Integrative Medicine, we unabashedly suggest allopathy if there is inconvenient or dangerous severity, such as when surgery or antibiotics are needed. For viruses, allopathy also does not usually have a quick response and the preventive use of vaccine is widely recommended.

Ayurveda and Traditional Chinese Medicine (and also homeopathy) are essential in the aftermath of the allopathic cure, though. The allopathic cure has side effects; the body's hardware and software are no longer correlated. Therefore, alternative medicine is a must to reestablish the physical-vital connections. Ignoring the aftermath treatment is a principal reason of diseases like multiple sclerosis and chronic fatigue—a general failure of vital-physical connection simultaneously for many organs.

Both Ayurveda and Traditional Chinese Medicine use food and natural herbs (which is naturopathy) to supply the missing creative software needed for healing.

Some of the herbs used have chemicals that resemble allopathic remedies. So there is a tendency to regard these herbs in reductionist ways, in terms of their chemical and physiological effect alone. But this misses the important vital energy aspect of herbal medicine. Whereas the herbs of the alternative medicine act on both physical and vital, when the active chemicals of such herbs are isolated, only their physiological effects remain, and we have lost the ability for vital software correction.

Does herbal medicine really work at the vital level, though? Is there a tangible effect? Western doctors collaborated with Chinese doctors to design a trial using a group of children suffering from the skin condition of eczema. The doctors prepared a "sham" tea made of a set of traditional herbs having nothing to do with the treatment of eczema and compared the effect of this with that of "real" tea made of the correct herbs prescribed according to the principles of Traditional Chinese Medicine. Half the group of children (randomly chosen) were given the real tea for an eight-week period, followed by a wash-out period of four weeks, and then another eight weeks of "sham" tea. The other half got the treatment in reverse order, sham tea first, then real tea. The results were dramatic. Whenever the children got the real tea, they saw a great improvement in their skin condition; whenever they got sham tea, their skin condition deteriorated drastically.

Like Ayurveda and unlike allopathic medicine (one treatment for all, more or less), treatments are individualized in Chinese medicine. This is because two individuals may both suffer from the same disease, say stomach ulcer, but the imbalances that gave rise to the ulcer may be very different in the two cases. By the same token, if two people have the same imbalances in the movement of vital energy, they can be treated in the same way, irrespective of their physical symptoms.

In this way, quantum science's confirmation of the concept of Ayurvedic dosha and heterogeneity of people is an excellent contribution to health and healing. The materialist approach can never bring about heterogeneity, can never provide individualized healthcare for people.

CHRONIC DISEASE

For chronic disease, Traditional Chinese Medicine has no extra concept, but Ayurveda does have the concept of tejas and pitta, which when treated in the quantum way, leads to an understanding.

Human beings evolved beyond animals with the help of the meaning processing mind. In the garden agricultural era of evolution, human beings discovered the archetype of love and this gave us the concept of family, which is based on the concept of love. The experience of maternal and romantic love was ritualized in the form of universal software in the collective unconscious. Other-love elevates the functioning of the heart chakra organs; self-love elevates the function of the navel chakra organs. This gave us new universal functional software for these organs.

Unfortunately, in the mental/rational current era, we messed it up. With the development of individuality to the extreme, many people suppress love (they avoid being vulnerable to another, mainly men); women, via necessity, culturally do not avoid love, but they are indoctrinated to avoid individuality. In this way, the dosha of pitta entered the scenario in a major way for both men and women.

Now to chronic disease. If you avoid other-love, you remain at the base level functioning for the immune system and it easily becomes malfunctional producing the vital stagnancy—energy block—at the heart chakra that is prerequisite for all sorts of chronic disease. Likewise, lack of self-love will produce energy block at the navel chakra. The mind also enters the game. A full discussion is given in Chapters 10 and 11 on mind-body disease.

THE FIVE-ELEMENT THEORY IS UNNECESSARY

Please note that in quantum Ayurveda the five-element theory is not needed. The idea of vital software, creativity, and conditioning eliminates the necessity.

The same is true for Traditional Chinese Medicine. Look at how, in view of what you have read, it is silly to invoke the five-element theory to explain how the lung develops phlegm-congestion when we contract common cold. Traditional Chinese Medicine developers theorized that the lung is a metal organ which has the capacity of holding water. With yin-yang imbalance, the lung loses some of its metallic property, cannot hold water anymore; the result is congestion. Notice how Ayurveda had already eliminated this kind of thinking by introducing the idea of *ama*, toxin accumulation in the body when the organs malfunction. Quantum theorizing—quantum science of Ayurveda—makes the explanation fool-proof.

chapter eight

PREVENTIVE MEDICINE LESSON I: BODY TYPES AND CORRESPONDING LIFESTYLES

In Chapter 7, we singled out a couple of the most telling characteristics for each dosha, purely for the purpose of distinguishing between them. But if you want to know which dosha or body type you belong to, a more detailed list is helpful, and one can be found in any standard book on Ayurveda. Deepak Chopra, Vasant Lad, and David Frawley all have written good books on the subject.

For mixed doshas, you will have a mixture of characteristics. The best way to know your dosha is to analyze your physical-vital development from childhood to adulthood. Here are some rules of thumb for determining your dosha:

- If you had an uneventful childhood with no physical or environmental challenges, you will have developed a very narrow spectrum of conditioned possibilities for your organ vital software to operate. This often develops the imbalance known as kapha dosha.
- If there were several challenges in childhood and you suffered from many diseases, you probably had a lot of vayu operating widening your spectrum of conditioned possibilities. This can

produce the imbalance known as vata dosha. Note, however that your susceptibility to childhood disease indicates inadequate existing vital software, most likely due to karma and an inherited kapha dosha.

- If you breezed through your development despite environmental challenges, this means you already had (from reincarnational inheritance) a good spectrum of conditioned vital possibilities to choose from, and that your vayu and ojas were adequate and balanced. In this case you end up with neither a kapha nor a vata dosha.
- In your early development, if you had the experience of being bullied or needing approval (for how you look, for example), you likely never awakened your navel chakra and consequently developed a lack of self-worth. A severe pitta dosha (perhaps from past karma) blocked you.
- In your teens, did you fall in love frequently and get into intimate heartful relationships? If you did, you had adequate tejas, and no pitta dosha. If, on the other hand, you were the independent kind, interested in sexual conquests rather than romance, you likely had developed a pitta dosha via past-life karma or in this life.
- If you are adventurous with food and prefer pungent and astringent flavors, that is an indication that tejas has been and is active in you. If however, you like pungent flavors, but your vital software cannot handle it and you suffer from frequent acidity, that is a sign of pitta dosha.
- Later in life, if you have environmental or lifestyle challenges and your body's vital software cannot handle it, and you need creativity but no creative outlet is available to you, that is a sure sign of your vata dosha being out of control.

Another rather effective way of identifying your dosha-prakriti is to analyze your personality. Are you a warm person? Then your heart chakra is active and you enjoy relationships. Pitta dosha is a likely diagnosis if you find yourself not exploring your heart much and not getting engaged in relationships much.

If others complain that you are a cold personality, you are either a kapha or a vata. If you are cold as well as dry, you are likely to be a vata type. Because of your vital hyperactivity, people will find you somewhat unapproachable.

If you are cold and moist, generally easy going, and easily approachable, you are a kapha type.

Caution: Traditional Ayurvedic books often ascribe cold, dry etc. to physical body attributes, like dry skin. No, they are about the vital body, how people feel to others.

Knowing your dosha and prakriti can be useful for more than just keeping you away from a gross overproduction of dosha imbalances. As the authors Robert E. Svoboda and Arnie Lade point out in their book *Tao and Dharma: Chinese Medicine and Ayurveda*, the efficacy of acupuncture can be greatly increased by modifying the usual technique according to the patient's dominant dosha imbalance.

DOSHA IMBALANCES

If you maintain your body according to your physical prakriti or base-level dosha or specific body type, then chances are good that you can breeze through life in good health. Problems arise when there is an imbalance, a disturbance in any of the doshas from this base level of prakriti. Generally, the imbalance is most likely to be in your own dominant body type—that is, a vata person is more likely to suffer from vata imbalance (overactive but ineffective vayu at the vital level).

However, there is no strict rule: You can be kapha person and still suffer from a pitta imbalance, not a kapha one. How can you tell if there is an imbalance beyond the level indicated in your prakriti? What causes these excess imbalances? One cause is seasonal change. And another, the major reason, is lifestyle.

DOSHA CONNECTIONS WITH THE SEASONS

There is a seasonal connection for the deviation of dosha imbalances from prakriti that can be predicated on the basis of the theory developed here. When the external environment is hot, as in the summer, that is the time for regeneration. Thus, tejas is attempted plentifully, let's say, by eating spicy, tasty food. If, however, the food is fast food or processed food—a spicy taco for example—then the attempt of invoking tejas is ineffective, the food does not nourish you, and tejas is ineffective, producing excess pitta.

When it is cold outside, it means either hibernation or the stability of ojas is needed. But again, if you reduce physical activity too much, excess ojas produces an imbalance of kapha. By the same token, if you over-engage in movements in an inattentive way, your vata will increase. If cold weather comes with dryness, the condition is ripe for a vata imbalance. If it is cold and wet (rain or snow), and all movement ceases, ojas dominates the vital body, and we end up with excess kapha.

Throughout the year, if you are observant, you can see how seasonal changes affect your dosha imbalances. On the East Coast of America, when the winter is cold and dry, many people use vayu in excess to enjoy movement, although it is so cold. They are risking developing vata aggravation.

But in early spring, when the weather turns cold and wet, it is time for many people to stop physical activity; that, too, opens the room for excess kapha imbalance, and one tends to catch cold (which, most often, is due to excess unbalanced kapha).

When it is hot and humid in the summer, you can easily notice, especially if you are a pitta type, that excess pitta is causing you problems with acidity. So in summertime we should all prefer cool foods and drinks to keep pitta down, and for pitta people, this is a must.

In general then, if your body type matches the environment, you have to be extra vigilant about keeping the imbalance from going out of control.

PREVENTIVE MEDICINE LESSON I

VATA IMBALANCE AND LIFESTYLE REMEDIES

If you are a vata person, but balanced in your prakriti, then you are cheerful, enthusiastic, and full of do-do-do energy. And why not? Whatever changes take place in your life situation, the reservoir of learned contexts of situational creativity at the vital level is able to reestablish your physical body homeostasis, provided your healing intention is intact.

But if you find that your expending energy is compromised by anxieties and worries, aches and pains, and sleeplessness, then ask (even if you are not predominantly vata): Is my vata still in balance as in my prakriti?

One scenario for vata imbalance is common to everyone: Vata tends to be aggravated with age. It is just part of the aging process; our consciousness is too busy using vayu for little adjustments of the body maintenance software. With this kind of vata aggravation, there is not much we can do. There is going to be some sleeplessness, some loss of memory (here is your chance to explore the experience of becoming an "absent-minded professor"), and some aches and pains. Even the appetite will not be like it used to be. When I myself (Amit) deal with these things at the ripe age of eighty-five at this writing, I always chuckle recalling a letter in which the great poet Rabindranath Tagore bitterly complained to a friend/devotee about his old-age problems.

But there are other scenarios. Suppose the change in your life situation is so drastic that the reservoir of those learned contexts of situational creativity you created with the vital creativity of vayu are not adequate to make the vital level adjustments required in a hurry. Your vayu is going to be overworked again, often causing a lot of vata fallout at the physical level. Situations like this arise in our life when we travel a lot, when we move our residence from one city to another, when we suffer through a divorce or the death of a spouse, or when we change jobs.

I (Amit) know this from personal experience. A couple of decades back, within the course of a year, I got divorced, I started courting another woman (whom I later married), I changed jobs, and I moved from one city to another much bigger city. On top of this, I got a research grant, so there was pressure of mental/intellectual accomplishments in a hurry that I had not encountered in years. And finally, I was already struggling with aggravated vata due to advancing age. Can you imagine the degree of vata aggravation all this caused? I was becoming so disoriented that during the year I had three auto accidents within a period of six months.

So what's the remedy from such unexpected lifestyle changes? Ayurvedic medicine suggests several tracks: proper diet; herbal remedies for vata aggravation; an environment of warmth and moisture; oil massage; certain hatha yoga exercises; the cleansing process of panchakarma that Valentina is so passionate about; and last, but not least, the practice of relaxation. The details of suitable diet and herbal remedies can be found in any good book on Ayurveda.

One advantage of Ayurvedic medicine is that once you learn the basics, applying it is mostly common sense, as you can see. So unless you neglect your imbalance for so long that the aggravation becomes severe (in which case the imbalance will manifest as the physical symptoms of what we normally call a disease), it is quite possible to use the above Ayurvedic recommendations as preventive medicine. You'll never need to go to a doctor.

In my own case, my usual regimen of yoga and meditation were unable to cope with the degree of vata aggravation, so I never did solve my vata imbalance problem while in the big city. Fortunately, aside from the auto accidents, I had no other physical disease due to the vata imbalance. Fortunately also, the movement of consciousness cooperated, and it was necessary to move away from the big city to my old, small-town habitat. Within six months, vata became balanced, mainly thanks to the relaxed lifestyle I could resume in my old habitat. I should mention, however, that my new wife helped in several ways: She provided me with a diet of fresh vegetarian food full of prana (called *sattvic* food in Ayurveda; see Chapter 13) and took long walks with me in nature, and with her I spent a lot less time ruminating and enjoyed much more laughter. (One problem concomitant with too much vata is too much mental work and the resulting tendency of taking yourself too seriously; you become full of—hot?—air.)

PITTA IMBALANCE AND LIFESTYLE REMEDIES

If you are a pitta person, even with some dosha obstruction, you probably exude vital creativity, and you are very intense. When pitta is balanced, you are able to handle your natural intensity with joy, and you obviously like being intense. But if the intensity is there and the joy is missing because of other life challenges, then chances are that your pitta has become unbalanced.

Do you see how it works? Pitta is a side effect of overworking tejas, fundamental creativity at the vital level. Tejas helps us build a good digestive system and maintain it with proper renewal as needed. But if the drive, do-do-do, is not balanced by relaxation that joy brings, the intensity becomes too much, the tejas is overworked without much desired result, and the effect is pitta imbalance.

A common scenario in which this happens occurs after age thirty before the transition to middle age. We have stopped physically growing by then, so the pressure on the digestive system and tejas at the vital level is considerably reduced. Unfortunately, though, the inertia of habit often keeps them going at the same level as at a younger age. This overworking of the tejas continues until we settle down in the second half of our lives. So in our thirties, pitta people have to accept a certain aggravation of pitta, which results in acidity and heartburn, the thinning of hair, a vulnerability to stress, and other things that take away the joy of intense vitality of creative life.

But there are also foolish ways to aggravate pitta such as overworking the digestive system unnecessarily with the improper kind of food. When we are young, our digestive fire is strong and it is considerably more intensified by eating hot and spicy food. The tejas of the food is all used up for a good cause—growing a healthy body. But when you don't need such intense digestive fire anymore, then overworking the system with unneeded tejas will produce avoidable pitta imbalance. If you fail to take notice, you will end up with chronic heartburn, even an ulcer.

Organization is not the forte of vitally creative people of the pitta type, and when such organizational demands are made, the system reacts with anger, frustration, and resentment, the expression of which requires tejas. The excessive use of tejas is the byproduct of excess pitta at the physical level. So emotional stress for adults in their thirties is a pitta aggravator. If you don't watch it, heart disease may result.

The remedy for pitta imbalance is moderation. Reduce the intake of stimulants like coffee. Meditate on loving kindness. Take long walks in nature; let that extra intensity be used up in the appreciation of archetypes like love, goodness, and beauty.

KAPHA IMBALANCE AND LIFESTYLE REMEDIES

As a kapha person, your strong point is strength and stability that endows you with a natural amount of generosity and affection to give to others. And this giving makes you happy. A kapha person is able to live a long, happy life. And yet a few glitches may arise.

In our childhood, the body of a healthy child is building itself; ojas is needed in abundance, and occasionally this will result in excess kapha. This gives a child susceptibility to catch colds, sore throats, sinus trouble, and so forth that will then continue as a predisposition for the rest of their life in an otherwise healthy existence. Remember though, you do not have to be a kapha person to contract this particular consequence of kapha imbalance.

But after our bodybuilding phase is over, excess ojas will have a tendency to produce obesity. This is the sign of kapha imbalance that may lead to other imbalances if not controlled.

On the emotional side, since our culture does not approve of obesity, insecurity results from kapha imbalance. If, in spite of this insecurity, one tries to be generous and giving, it will produce clinging and contraction of consciousness instead of expansion.

On the physical side, obesity puts too much stress on the heart and leads to hypertension and difficulty in breathing.

Still another scenario is a faulty diet, heavy in sweets for example. One manifestation of this route to kapha imbalance is diabetes.

Whereas vata imbalance requires a ho-hum life, kapha imbalance requires the opposite: more stimulation and variety to shake up the inertia. Controlling kapha imbalance also requires weight control, avoidance of sweets, and rigorous exercise routine.

YOGA AND AYURVEDA: HOW TO DEVELOP THE BEST PRACTICE FOR YOUR DOSHA BODY TYPE

No two people are the same. In Ayurveda, constitution—prakriti—is based on the predominant dosha, the body type. Your constitution affects many aspects of your life—from what you look like to how you deal with challenges, and everything in between.

As your constitution is such a major influence, understanding it is a powerful way to develop an effective practice. We'll take a look at the strengths and weaknesses of each dosha and discuss how you can use these to reach your highest potential through yoga and meditation.

If you're not sure which body type you are, you can go to an Ayurvedic doctor and get a full consultation. An experienced practitioner can pinpoint your exact constitution based on your pulse, tongue, eyes, fingernails, and other details. Otherwise, you can take an online quiz to get a basic idea of what you're dealing with. These are readily available.

Let's recap. According to Ayurveda, your dosha must be considered when you decide what you should eat, when and how much you should sleep, what exercise you should do, and what your yoga practice should be like.

The point of being aware of your dosha constitution is not to try to create an equal balance of all three doshas in your being, since this is not natural for most people. Instead, you want to restore the balance of doshas according to your prakriti, the natural proportion you ended with as you grew up.

Now that you understand your constitution and tendencies, let's take a look at how to develop a yoga practice suited to your dosha in order to counteract your imbalances and make the most out of your natural strengths.

RECOMMENDATIONS FOR KAPHA-DOMINANT PEOPLE

In kapha-dominant people, the inner fire (*agni*—the supramental archetypes of change) tends to run low. This can result in sluggishness, drowsiness, poor digestion, low energy, and excess body weight. To counter this, choose a practice that is active and dynamic.

The good news for kapha people is that you probably have a lot of vitality in potentiality—much more than people for whom pitta or vata is dominant. This means that although your energy might seem "heavy" and more difficult to get moving, once it starts moving you'll have a lot of power to support it.

Surya namaskara: Sun salutations are dynamic and increase heat in the body, making them very effective for kapha people. By cultivating resonance with the sun, considered the source of all life activity on Earth, sun salutations balance out the cold, inert nature of kapha.

Manipura (navel chakra)-enhancing asanas: Any asana that activates the manipura chakra will help burn off excess kapha. Many manipura asanas (for example, Trikonasana) are also very physically demanding, which is healthy for stimulating a slow metabolism and doesn't allow for over-relaxation in the practice.

Kapha people are generally calm and steady, which easily carries over into meditation. However, they tend towards dullness and sleepiness, and they are more likely to get stuck in patterns. There's a danger of the practice becoming just another habit. Keep yourself fresh and alert in meditation by doing some yoga or exercise beforehand. It helps to meditate in a place with a lot of light.

Be very vigilant about dullness. Maintain a firm, upright posture, with a commitment to staying clear. If you get drowsy, focus on your inhalation for a few breaths, visualize a bright light, or even open your eyes for a minute.

Experimenting with new techniques and constantly reminding yourself of your motivation can help keep the spark in your practice. Devotional practices like prayer, chanting, or singing bhajans are also very good.

RECOMMENDATIONS FOR PITTA-DOMINANT PEOPLE

For pitta people, the main challenge in yoga is the excess energy active in the body. This type will often love a more dynamic practice, with lots of sun salutations and moving quickly from pose to pose, but this is exactly what they don't need.

Since it can be difficult for fiery people to go directly into stillness, they can start their practice by channeling their intense energy in other ways gradually.

Go through a few rounds of *surya namaskara*, but with the emphasis on awareness, observing the inner stillness even while the body is in motion. Gradually decrease the speed of the performance and take longer pauses between rounds to center in the Heart. As the breathing pattern slows, the vital energies and the mind will also settle down.

Once some of the excess energy has been burned off, you can go into a practice that emphasizes grounding and stability.

Include a lot of forward bends and poses that don't require much effort. These engage the parasympathetic nervous system, or the "rest and digest" aspect of the nervous system (as opposed to fight-or-flight, which activates the sympathetic nervous system). The balance between the parasympathetic nervous system and the sympathetic nervous system is important.

Try to deeply relax in every asana. Hold them for a long time and feel stillness in the organs of your body. Even if you feel the urge to move, witness this impulse and absorb the energy without reacting.

Pitta people have fire inside. They can be very intense and focused, and dullness is usually not a problem. There are two main challenges that pitta-dominant people might run into in meditation.

First, they may have trouble relaxing. Unharnessed fire energy brings a lot of physical restlessness. Until the body is settled, it will be difficult for the mind to become calm. That's why for pitta people it's good to start with a more dynamic practice before settling into meditation.

Second, the pitta personality is competitive, perfectionist, driven, and highly active. This is a double-edged sword in wholeness practice. It's great to have a lot of passion and intensity. They say in the Jewish Kabbalah that the *Shekhinah* (the feminine face of God) gets bored with those who worship Her just correctly and within the rules: She wants people to be on fire with Divine Love.

Pitta people aren't ones to slack off in their practice or let it turn into a routine. However, when their drive comes from the ego, from a need to be the best or to make something happen, it becomes yet another barrier in the journey toward health and happiness. It can get you stuck more firmly in the idea of being the doer, developing an inflated spiritual ego, and make you prone to contraction of consciousness rather than expansion.

So, become friends with the idea that letting go doesn't mean giving up your fiery nature. Cultivate surrender, a deeper octave of relaxation where activity is maintained while the sense of acting is dissolved.

Consecrate before every practice and, afterwards, dedicate its fruits to the benefit of the entire Universe, as a reminder that your practice isn't for yourself. "I do this practice with love and harmony. I consecrate it to use for the world and myself to truth."

Practice blindfolded or alone if you're always comparing yourself to others. Finally, be compassionate towards yourself and humble in acknowledging your limits. Rest when you need to.

RECOMMENDATIONS FOR VATA-DOMINANT PEOPLE

Vata people can be extremely active thinkers—the do-do-do vital hyperactivity extends to the mental as well, with a tendency to produce attention problems. As the vata moves, so does the mind, and it moves fast. This can make it hard to stay focused and relaxed during yoga.

To settle down into the practice, it helps to work with the breath. Stay constantly aware of the breath, especially the way it moves in your abdomen, and feel how it slows as you relax into each asana.

Give plenty of time for the immobility of the body (*kaya sthairyam* in Sanskrit) to phase-in the asana, connecting deeply to your body and feeling the stillness in every organ.

If you're stuck in the mind, going into the body will pull you out of mental loops and into the present moment, since the body is your stable reference point.

Predominance of the air and ether elements (mental and spiritual) mean that vata people often cannot hold onto vitality, which is fickle. This manifests as physical weakness and low energy. Vata people also often feel ungrounded, like they are lost in a colorful swirl of thoughts and plans and ideas, and somehow their connection to the concrete reality they inhabit disappears.

Practicing a lot of grounding asanas helps with both of these problems. Asanas for *muladhara* (*Badrasana* will work for this one as well) will both increase physical energy and bring mental peace, stability, and security. Best of all is to meditate and practice muladhara asanas while on the bare ground, in order to directly absorb vital energy from Earth's biota.

Mental agitation is the main vata challenge in meditation. If you seem to spend most of your meditation time chasing around your thoughts, try starting your yoga sessions with a practice called Capturing the Uncaught Mind, or *tratakam*, by holding your attention on a candle flame; walking meditation also can calm the mind.

Come back as much as you can to a sense of stillness and relaxation in the body. Being aware of the pauses in the breathing cycle is a potent tool for calming the mind throughout the practice of meditation and yoga. Sink fully into every pause, enjoying the feeling of timelessness.

Vata loves change, excitement, and new things. Vata people, therefore, are always eager to move on to new techniques and explore other practices. This is great, because vata people don't get stuck in being bored with their current practice. However, it makes it hard to go deep into anything. It is said that if you want water, don't dig fifty shallow wells. Just dig one deep well. It's good to keep learning, living with a sense of curiosity and wonderment. But you should also be able to go deep.

I (Valentina) recommend choosing a practice or technique that resonates with you and sticking with it every day, at least for six months or so, until you can really see where it is taking you. Along with that, you can feel free to experiment and try new things, but your practice will have a backbone to support the new additions.

INTERNAL HYGIENE: PANCHAKARMA

In Ayurveda, great emphasis is put on the periodic cleansing of the systems of our body to cleanse them of excess humors, also called *ama*, that occur due to the imbalances of vata, pitta, and kapha. For example, pitta imbalance will create ama in the intestines. Ama can be dealt with through periodic cleansing of the affected organs. Panchakarma consists of five such cleansing procedures: therapeutic sweating; nasal cleansing with or without herbs; purgation of the stomach and intestines achieved through herbs or enemas, oil massage; and bloodletting. Panchakarma requires the supervision of a trained Ayurvedic physician.

chapter nine

PREVENTIVE MEDICINE LESSON 2:
THE QUANTUM SCIENCE OF THE CHAKRAS

When we experience emotion, there is not only a mental thought but also a feeling that accompanies it. What do we feel? We feel the movement of vital energy accompanying the emotion. But where in the body do we feel the feeling component of our emotions?

A connoisseur of feeling will say that it depends on the emotion as well as who you are. If you are an intellectual, it is likely that you will only feel vital energy in the head. When we are being intellectual, the vital energy goes to the brow chakra.

If you are not predominantly an intellectual, then you will recognize other places in the body where you feel your energy going. The most familiar of these places is of course, the heart chakra, the place where you feel romantic energy. Can you remember the first time you realized you were in love? Close your eyes and remember that moment right now; soon you will feel the surge of energy in your heart chakra (felt as a throb, a tingle, warmth, or just expansion). This is why people read romance novels or watch mushy, heart-warming movies—to revisit these feelings. They (women mostly) like the surge of energy (warmth) in their heart chakra.

In contrast, when people (men mostly) watch sex and violence on

TV, no doubt their negative emotional brain circuits get involved, but there are vital energy movements in the first three low chakras as well. This activity may help people to feel grounded.

When we feel good about ourselves, we feel an energy boost in our navel chakra; if we feel insecure, we feel energy going out of that chakra: butterflies in the stomach. We feel rooted when the energy moves into the root chakra, but when the energy drains out of there, we feel fear.

The sex chakra is where the vital energy appears when we feel amorous. Viagra may help a man get erections when he is old, but there is no replacement of the vitality required to enjoy sexuality. This why people feel dissatisfied with Viagra sex: drug-induced erections may not come with vitality in the form of sexual energy. The mechanics are there, but the vitality may lack; Viagra sex is mostly mental.

After sex, or after a good meal, the energy rises to the heart chakra; no doubt the women of old knew this, since they often asked their husbands for household needs or money after sex or after food intake. Ever heard the phrase, "the way to a man's heart is through the stomach"?

When we are nervous about giving a speech, our throat seems to dry up; this is because vital energy has moved out of the throat chakra, and the physical effect is that a high dose of adrenaline inhibits the salivary glands. Our mental interpretation of the vital block at the throat influences the adrenal gland via psycho-neuro-gastrointestinological connections. On the other hand, when you are communicating well, feel the throat chakra. You will enjoy the vibes there; we all do.

When we concentrate on something intellectual, our eyebrows focus and we can feel heat in the midpoint of our eyebrows, at the brow chakra. Right behind it is the prefrontal cortex where our intellectual thoughts are processed. The further opening (a term used to signify awakening) of this chakra makes us more open to intuitive thoughts and creative insights as if a new way of visioning, a "third eye," has come about. In India, when people do spiritual work it creates a time for a great many intuitive experiences, and the third eye becomes so hot that people use sandalwood paste to soothe it. You may have seen Indian women wear a *bindi* on their forehead; the reason is to calm a woman's sensitivity to intuition.

So, once again, chakras are places in our physical bodies where we feel vital energy localized when we are experiencing an emotion.

THE QUANTUM SCIENCE OF THE CHAKRAS

If you examine Figure 3, you will notice that each of the chakras is situated near one or more important organs of our body. This has been noted since millennia and is a clue toward the scientific understanding of chakras.

Remember our earlier discussion of liturgical fields? The vital body liturgical fields provide the blueprint for the epigenetic vital software that program organ functions. Rupert Sheldrake discovered the original idea of liturgical fields (aka morphogenetic fields) but did not see their connection to feelings. I (Amit) did not know about the chakras much either until I attended a transpersonal psych conference and listened to a talk on chakra psychology. That talk led synchronistically to the combination of these two ideas: Chakras are those places in your physical body where consciousness simultaneously actualizes the vital and the physical in the process of which the software programs are run, organ functions take place, the correlated liturgical fields move, and you feel that movement in the form of vital energy.

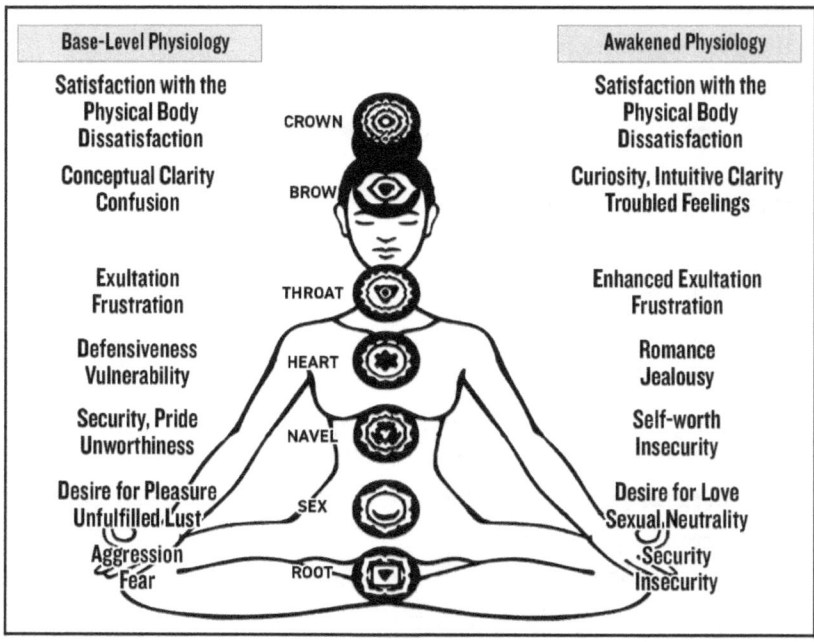

Figure 11. The chakras and their associated feelings change when the brow, heart, and navel selves awaken. The feelings associated with base-level physiology are shown on the left; feelings associated with the awakened physiology are shown on the right. For each chakra, the upper feeling is the positive one experienced when the chakra-organs are functioning well; the lower feeling indicates the negativity experienced when the chakra-organ functions are disrupted.

Here, then, is a chakra-by-chakra description of the physiology of the physical organs at the chakra and the associated feelings (Figure 11) for base-level physiology:

The Root Chakra: The organ physiology is elimination, a crucial component of maintenance of the body called catabolism. The organs which express the function are the kidneys, bladder, large intestine, rectum, anus, and, most importantly, the adrenal gland. The feelings are feelings of (selfish) rootedness and survival-oriented competitiveness when the energy moves in and fear when the energy moves out. Via evolution, the control of this chakra is taken over by the brain amygdala which gives the fear (flight) or aggressiveness (fight) response.

The Sex Chakra: The vital body function is reproduction. The reproductive organs—uterus, ovaries, prostate, and testes, etc.—all contribute to the reproductive function. The feelings are those of sexuality and amour when energy moves in; when energy is outgoing, the feeling is of (unfulfilled) lust. Once again, the control is in the amygdala of the midbrain through the testes and the ovary glands.

The Navel Chakra: The organ function is maintenance (anabolism) and the organs involved are the stomach and small intestine, liver, gall bladder, and pancreas. With upsurge of energy at this chakra, the feeling is pride; when energy moves out, the feelings are anger, unworthiness, resentment, etc. all derived from basic insecurity. These negative feelings are contributed by the brain's amygdala via the gland of pancreas.

When children develop autonomy, they awaken their navel chakra and experience self-worth.

The Heart Chakra: The body function is self-distinction between the "me" and the "not me" of the thymus gland of the immune system. The feeling is defensiveness when energy moves in and vulnerability when energy moves out. But of course many people feel romance at the heart when energy moves in. When energy moves out, these people feel loss, grief, hurt, and sometimes jealousy. What gives?

We need to elaborate: Why is romance felt at the heart chakra when these romantics meet the appropriate partner? Because now their "me" is extended to include the partner, that's why. Somehow the immune system's distinction of me vs. not me and of defensiveness is gone. Why? because the immune system is momentarily suspended. And when that happens, the heart awakens into a quantum mode of coherent movement and is capable of a new function—romance. This is the romantic love that people feel.

The Throat Chakra: The physiological function is making sounds of expression. The organs are the lungs, the throat and its vocal chords, the speech organs, the hearing organs, and the thyroid gland. The associated feelings are the exultation of freedom (of speech) when energy moves in and frustration when energy moves out. (You may recognize why freedom of speech is considered so important in our culture although true freedom is freedom of choice.)

The Third Eye: The physiological function is rational thinking for which the organ is the prefrontal cortex right at the back of the forehead. The associated feelings are clarity of understanding when energy moves in and confusion with depletion of energy. With further opening, this is the chakra that funnels intuitive energy associated with archetypal experiences. The associated feeling that initiates archetypal exploration is curiosity; when the curiosity is properly addressed, we feel satisfaction; when the curiosity does not end in success, we feel despair.

The Crown Chakra: The physiological function is body-knowledge and body-image for which the physical organ is the parietal lobe. Sense of identity with the physical body comes from this chakra. When you look at a mirror and like your body image, energy is coming into the chakra giving you a feeling of okayness about yourself; if you don't like what you see in the mirror, the energy quits and you feel distraught.

Figure 11 shows the chakras and the associated feelings when the chakras are awakened to quantum functioning and some of the organ physiology is elevated.

Of crucial significance is the fact that there is an endocrine gland associated with each of the chakras. The endocrine glands communicate with the brain for the chakras in the body, including the heart. In this way, through this "psycho-neuro-immunological" connection as well as through the autonomic nervous system, the mind gets control over the vital energies at the body chakras after the initial response is over and the neocortex gets into the act.

DISEASES AT THE CHAKRAS

In her book, *Frontiers of Health: How to Heal the Whole Person*, physician Christine Page unabashedly classifies many organ diseases as nonnormal energy movement at one chakra or another. Here is a sample of the diseases that Page lists (we have altered the list slightly) as possible if energy movement goes awry at the chakras:

Root Chakra: constipation, hemorrhoids, colitis, diarrhea, etc.
Sex Chakra: impotence, vaginismus; prostrate disease for males and disease of the female reproductive system for females.
Navel Chakra: irritable bowel syndrome; diabetes, peptic and gastric ulcer, liver disease, hiatus hernia.
Heart Chakra: heart disease, auto-immune disease, cancer, maybe dementia.

Cancer is listed as a heart chakra disease for good reason. Cancer cells are abnormal cells and in principle, the immune system should be able to detect them and eliminate them. One reason cancer occurs is because of immune system malfunction, and therefore, cancer may be related with nonnormal movement of vital energy at the heart. Cancer can develop in any organ due to the immune system's failure at that site; subsequently, cancer can spread to any and all organs, a process called metastasizing. Curiously, even after spreading, it always retains the character of the original cancer. This shows that local aggravation adds to the immune system malfunction, giving rise to the cancer of that organ. For example, smoking along with a lack of love will cause cancer of the lung. People who have love can escape cancer even though they smoke. This is not to justify the nasty and dangerous habit of smoking because, in our experience, not many smokers continue to love adequately for very long in their relationship unless they pay attention. And of course, there are also emphysema and other serious breathing diseases to consider.

Why does the immune system malfunction when heart energy—love—is absent? Love is when the immune system's defensive function is temporarily suspended. So the immune system must have ongoing momentary suspension adding up to a rest period just as our neo-cortex uses sleep to get rest. This needing rest has to do with the fact that there is a self-identity associated with the heart chakra as well as with the neocortex.

Throat Chakra: Over- or under-active thyroid; asthma; sore throat; ear disease

Brow Chakra: Migraine and tension headaches; eye disease; mind-brain diseases like depression and schizophrenia; Alzheimer's disease

Crown Chakra: Apotemnophilia, somatoparaphrenia, anorexia, and bulimia

Apotemnophilia is a peculiar disease in which the patient expresses desire for the amputation of a healthy body part. Such patients would say, "I'd rather cut off my left arm." Somatoparaphrenia is a similar disease that arises when the right parietal lobe is damaged by a stroke. The patient does not want his left upper arm anymore. (For more information, see V. S. Ramachandran's book, *The Tell-Tale Brain*).

Very briefly, chakra medicine consists of complementing the treatment of the physical symptoms (through allopathy), addressing the pranic imbalance (through Ayurveda, Chinese medicine, or homeopathy) with psychological work on the mindset, and psychic healing through direct pranic infusion by a pranic healer to the affected chakra.

The good news is that almost everyone can be a pranic healer, for we all have psychic ability to that extent. In the West, not many people are familiar with feeling the movement of prana, but it is easily learned. A simple exercise for understanding how prana works is to rub your palms together and then bring them apart by about half an inch in the East Indian style of greeting called "namaste" (which, by the way means, "I greet you from the place where you and I are one"). You will feel tingles that are not from blood circulation or nerve impulses: This is the movement of prana in the skin. You can amplify the tingling by outstretching your arms (Taoist style), opening your palms to the canopy of the sky and inviting all the healing chi and the universal chi from extraterrestrial biota that the universe is willing to send you. Now your palms are energized and you are ready to give pranic healing to a friend.

Chakra medicine benefits from concomitant chakra psychology, in which a therapist tries to correct the mindset that is causing the energy imbalance at the chakra. For example, breast cancer may indicate a lack of self-love as well as a lack of other types of love, and psychotherapy can help with rekindling love.

Q & A

What do we really mean by "activation of chakras"? Is it paying attention to them and experiencing feelings?
Authors: The organs go on functioning as determined potentialities. Activation is collapsing these movements into actuality and experiencing the associated vital feeling. This would be a positive feeling.

What does "vitalizing of chakras" mean? Is it the same as in the question above?
Authors: Not quite. We vitalize a chakra when we bring creative response either to a vital nonlocal stimulus from another living being (such as a loved one) or to an intuition (such as looking at a flower and intuiting its beauty). You can think of the latter as a kind of tuning in, similar to resonance.

What does movement of energy from one chakra to another mean? Is it like energy being depleted at one place and enhanced at another chakra? If so, like the physical energy, does the vital energy also have law of conservation?
Authors: When we breathe, as we inhale, we bring oxygen and the organ functions more vigorously and as the oxygen moves in, another organ starts functioning vigorously, etc. You can think of this as a movement of vital energy, vitality from one chakra to another using known pathways, the meridians or nadis. Similar movements can be effected

by moving your activated palms from chakra to chakra. Yeah, energy is being depleted in one place (being brought to the default level) and enhanced in another in the process. However unlike physical energy, there is no conservation law when we are creative. Subtle energy is infinite; there is no need for a conservation law. Via resonance (see Chapter 4) we bring new archetypal energy all the time, if we are so sensitive.

What does the blocking and unblocking of the chakras mean? And how does that block happen in the first place?
Author: We exist and our organs continue to function when we are alive, so the vital energy at all chakras need to be "moving" because, otherwise, how else will the body function? When energy is blocked, the organ is not functioning according to its usual determined potentiality mode. Pay attention next time your bowel does not clear; you can easily feel the resulting loss of vitality. This is the reason Ayurveda puts such big emphasis on regular bowel movements.

When sexual energy is blocked, you will have no interest in sex, which is a common happening for many women, and even some men, after a few years of marriage or after a child or two, and it may become difficult to motivate ourselves to be creative.

It is the contention of this book that an energy block in the root chakra is responsible for root chakra chronic diseases like irritable bowel syndrome. A blocked navel chakra is responsible for Type II diabetes; a blocked heart chakra can cause cancer; and a brow chakra block can bring on Alzheimer's.

chapter ten

QUANTUM MIND: MEANING, EMOTIONS, AND MEDICINE

Mind-body medicine does not make sense until you realize that it is not a consequence of mind over body, but instead is a consequence of consciousness over body. Both body (in the form of the brain) and mind are quantum possibilities of consciousness. In the event of a collapse of the waves of possibility, consciousness uses the mind to give meaning to both external and internal possibilities actualized in the brain. Simultaneously, consciousness uses the neurons of the brain to make representations (memories) of the mental meaning. If the meaning that mind gives misguided by brain memory for an otherwise meaning-neutral stimulus is disharmonious, taking you away from ease, watch out: Mind-body disease may result. But consciousness also has the capacity to shift the context of mental meaning, so healing also is within its purview. This is mind-body healing.

EMOTIONAL STRESS: EVIDENCE FOR MIND-BODY DISEASE

First, we need to define some terms. A stressor is an outside agent, which can be a death in the family, a math problem, an exam, a boring job, etc. A stress is how a person reacts or responds to a stressor. This means that, once again, what mental meaning we put to the stressor, and how we mentalize—that is, give meaning that is often exaggerated or even wrong—the feeling associated with our reaction to the stressor.

In a given culture, meanings become somewhat fixated and the stress associated with many common stressors produce similar stress responses in most people. We can talk about an average response. The researcher Richard Rahe measured such average stress in "life-change units," or LCUs—the degree of life adjustments a stressor requires. For example, in Rahe's study, a minor illness has a stress level of 25 LCUs, whereas in the death of a spouse, the count goes up to 105 LCUs.

Even a seemingly simple stress like an exam can kill a person. More people die of heart attacks on Monday than on any other day, thanks to the so-called "black Monday syndrome." Monday is the day when people return from a relaxed weekend and fantasize about how stressful the workweek is going to be, or how boring or difficult and so forth, and their hearts succumb to the stress. It is mentalization that kills people.

There is now at least some preliminary evidence that stress can cause disease of the gastrointestinal system as well. One example is stomach ulcer, regardless of some allopaths claiming that ulcer is caused by a bacterium. Stress can cause severe diseases of the respiratory system like asthma, and of the immune system, such as cancer, heart disease, and autoimmune diseases in which the immune system attacks the body's own cells. The organs in the body are not independent of the mind-brain duo.

PSYCHO-NEURO-IMMUNOLOGY: THE BRAIN-MIND TAKEOVER OF THE CHAKRAS IN THE BODY

Imagine that following a certain stressor, you are angry and very upset. Your brain is mapping your angry thoughts. But can your brain communicate its maps to your body, specifically to the immune system?

The organs of the immune system, including the thymus gland, are also called lymphoid organs because they produce lymphocytes, the all-important white blood cells that are the mediators of the immune response of the body. The initial production of lymphocytes takes place in the bone marrow. One set of them, the T cells, inhabit the thymus gland early in their development and become the conveyor of the me-and-not-me distinction. Lymphocytes travel throughout the body in the form of small armies that are kept alert in the lymph nodes and the spleen. It is via these lymphatic organs that the immune system's job of distinguishing me-and-not-me continues even after the thymus gland semi-retires at about age sixteen.

The immune system is what defends us, the body, against intruders: viruses, bacteria, any foreign not-me object. Initially, this seems quite independent of what the brain does. But surprisingly, a neurologist at the University of Rochester discovered that the immune system organs have nerves all over them; it is quite plausible that the immune system communicates with the brain. But why? The plot thickened in 1981 when neurophysiologist Robert Ader discovered that the immune system could be conditioned using the same procedure as mental conditioning.

Let's consider the classic experiment of Ader that prompted him to coin the word "psychoneuroimmunology." Ader was working on a Pavlovian conditioning experiment of teaching rats the aversion of saccharine-flavored water. The standard practice was to correlate the rats' drinking of water with the injection of a drug (psychophosphamide) that induces nausea and vomiting. Rats quickly learned to associate the sweet water with the nausea. After the conditioning, the rats would experience nausea only with sweet water, and the drug was not needed any more. But there was a peculiar complication. The rats also seemed to have learned to die as a result of drinking sweetened water: The psychophosphamide was inducing a suppression of the immune system. The conditioning not only taught the rats to simulate, upon drinking sweet water, the nauseating effect of the drug, but also to suppress the immune system. It was the suppression of the immune system that made the rats prone to disease and death.

Experiments soon followed even at the human level. One of the first such studies correlated the infection rate of sailors while on board of a ship with their actual life events. The sailors who were the most unhappy as a result of their life events were also found to have the highest rate of infection. Perceived negative meaning produces stress, which produces infection via the suppression of the immune system—a clear case of psychoneuroimmunology.

Stress produced by a spouse's death can lead to reduced functioning of the immune system by reducing its arsenal of killer T cells compromising defence from bacteria and viruses. There is little doubt that grief is a factor contributing to breast cancer among women.

Don't get too hung up with all this negative talk about how stress affects the immune system negatively. There is also the Mother Theresa effect. In a study at Harvard University, students were shown a film of Mother Teresa lovingly taking care of destitute, dying people. The film increased the students' immune system functioning as evidenced by the increase of an immune enhancement marker (increase of salivary IgA). This is psychoneuroimmunology, too. Love is an antidote for immune system stressors.

MOLECULES OF EMOTION

What mediates the interaction of the immune system with the brain? In the 1970s, neuroscientist/pharmacologist Candace Pert and others discovered that the brain secretes certain molecules called neuropeptides that help mediate analgesia, hormonal changes, and other responses to stress and resulting illnesses (see Pert's book, *Molecules of Emotion*). Among the neuropeptides, perhaps the most famous are the endorphins, which attach to specific receptor sites in the brain and the body (interestingly enough, fitting as in a lock-and-key mechanism). How the endorphins (or the lack of them) can alter our experience of pain (or pleasure) has been well covered in the popular press. For example, take the case of hot chili pepper which, like many people, we the present authors like. Why is hot pepper pleasurable—that is, allowing one to experience pain mixed with pleasure—when, according to its molecular composition, its spicy hot flavor should give us only pain? The answer is endorphins. If you eat a hot pepper along with taking an endorphin blocker, what you will feel is pure, unadulterated pain.

The neuropeptide connection is two-way: Brain endorphins connect to the immune system, and the immune system molecule thymosine connects to the brain. Similar two-way connections have been established between the brain and the endocrine system as well—psycho-neuroendocrinology.

MENTAL GUNAS

The usual approach of proponents of mind-body medicine is to first demonstrate with data that the mind does cause disease; then demonstrate, through a discussion of psychoneuroimmunology and psycho-neuroendocrinology, how the mind affects the body; and lastly go into the healing techniques of mind-body medicine. But with quantum science, we can do better.

The straightforward approach does not explain why not everybody contracts mind-body disease or why the response to stress is not universal. There is data showing that people who are optimistic, are committed to their work and have control over it, look at stressors as challenges to be overcome, and do not suffer from the ill effects of stress. There are also mentally lazy people among us who somehow breeze through life without feeling stress.

The fact is that there is individuality in our mental response to the stressors. Just as the unbalanced use of creativity and conditioning and the vital gunas of vayu and ojas create certain doshas in the physical body, there exist certain mental gunas (qualities) whose unbalanced use also creates doshas in the brain.

There are three mental gunas, each given a Sanskrit name: *sattva*, which is usually translated as the quality of illumination; *rajas*, denoting the empire building tendency of the raja or king; and *tamas*, which means darkness, denoting inertia. In quantum science, sattva is the capacity for fundamental creativity, rajas is the capacity for situational creativity, and tamas is the tendency for maintaining status quo, inertia. Note that for creativity, do-be-do-be-do, we need both the creative qualities and the quality of conditioning. In this way, gunas should be in balance.

MIND-BRAIN DOSHAS AND MIND-BODY DISEASES

The science of Ayurvedic medicine is based on this idea: unbalanced application of the gunas (qualities) at the vital level gives rise to doshas (defects)—kapha, vata, pitta—at the physical-vital organ level. Thus, we should look for the analogs of the vital doshas created by the mind via the childhood misuse of its qualities or gunas. And since the mind is only correlated with the neocortex, and these doshas will belong to the cortical brain, let's call them mind-brain doshas.

It is not hard to see what these mind-brain doshas are. An unbalanced use of mental sattva, produces insensitivity to the true meaning of intuitions, and creates the intellectual: one who uses new contexts (problems) only for more rational thinking, not to look at creative solutions. A side effect of insensitivity to intuition is insensitivity to feelings in the body as well; in other words, an intellectual tends to become detached from the body.

A Sufi story beautifully reminds us of this danger. The perennial hero of such wisdom tales, Mulla Nasruddin, a boatman in this story, is taking a pundit in his boat to a certain destination. As soon as they start their journey, the pundit starts giving Nasruddin a sample of his knowledge—in this case, grammar. But Nasruddin is bored and does not try to hide it. He begins yawning. The pundit gets irritated and says, "If you don't know grammar, half of your life is wasted." Nasruddin lets the comment pass. After a while, the boat develops a problem and begins to capsize. Nasruddin asks the pundit if he knows how to swim, and the pundit replies in the negative, adding that the idea of physical exercise has always bored him. Says Mulla Nasruddin, "In that case, all of your life is wasted. The boat is sinking."

Unbalanced use of mental rajas gives rise to short attention span and hyperactivity at the physical brain level. Hyperactive people live a do-do-do lifestyle, being always tuned to mental accomplishments—the outcome rather than the process. Attention deficit hyperactive disorder, which is all too common in the age of the Internet, is an extreme case of this mind-brain dosha.

Unbalanced mental inertia, or tamas, gives rise to mental nonengagement with new stimulations of the brain, a basic lethargy of the ego to engage in new mental learning not to be confused with genetically inherited mental retardation. This may happen due to parental neglect in creating a sufficiently stimulating environment. It may also happen due to a mismatch of past-life propensities with the stimulations available in the child's environment.

Autism is in part due to a lack of mirror neuron response in a child. Mirror neurons are built-in circuits in the brain that imitate other people's behavioral responses to a stimulus. This is how negative emotions and even some positive expressions, like laughing, become contagious. Lack of mirror neurons makes a child lack in the usual socio-cultural response. This part of the cause of autism could be genetic in origin.

There is also a developmental contribution that goes back to the fetus in the mother's womb. In late pregnancy, some women get depressed. Since the fetus is nonlocally correlated with the mother, the mother's depression can affect the baby's potentialities, which are collapsed after the baby is born. In this way, the emotional disconnect that we see in autistic children can develop.

We believe there is even a contribution of reincarnation to autism. The mismatch of past-life propensities with environment contributes to autism. The child simply becomes disinterested and surrenders to the ever-present guna of tamas and develops mental apathy.

Indeed, a study published in the journal *The Lancet* shows that if parents are trained to try to communicate during the early stages autistic children's development, the children's communication abilities improve and repetitive behavior is reduced, suggesting a reduction of mental slowness. Clearly, parents' attention keeps the children interested and helps overcome the effect of environmental mismatch with their karmic propensities.

Although these mind-brain doshas reside in the brain, they do govern our attitude toward all emotions—the ones from the brain as well as those from the body. Of people of the three doshas, only the mentally "lazy" avoids the mind-brain duo and lives in the body—not only in the three lower chakras, but also in the heart. People of the other two doshas "mentalize" their feelings regularly, giving wrong meaning to feelings. People of predominant intellectuality will suppress the perceived emotions and may suffer from chronic depression as a result. People of dominant rajasic dosha—hyperactivity—on the other hand, are the expressive kind and are easily irritable and prone to quick anger and hostility in their reaction to stress. Hyperactivity is also associated with anxiety. Hollywood movies such as *Forest Gump* seem to portray the idea that only the simpleton can be happy, can be nice to others. There may be some truth to that.

RESPONSE TO EMOTION: EXPRESSION

How do you respond to emotions? In the West, especially in America, there is strong cultural conditioning against expressing emotions. Expressing emotions is considered a sign of weakness and hence, almost universally, Western men have traditionally learned to suppress emotions as they grow up. Whereas for women who were formerly recognized as the "weaker sex," the cultural conditioning against expressing emotions is not as deep (this is now changing due to women demanding equality).

Nevertheless, not all Western men engage in suppressing emotions. In fact, some narcissistic men tend to indulge in expressing emotions, not having the usual social constraint of defending one's persona.

You can see such people everywhere today because of, seemingly, an epidemic in narcissism. Under emotional stress, these people have well-recognized responses of short temper or irritability. We can see the connection with mind-brain doshas here with dominant hyperactivity. This is especially true when excess hyperactivity, out of balance with one's nature, develops.

If one is fortunate enough to always have a family member or friend or even a sycophant to allow the ventilation of emotions, this other person can help dissipate the negative impact of the emotional expressions. In traditional societies as in India, this used to be the general rule and still is to a considerable extent, so the health impact of emotive expression is relatively minor. But now it is all changing.

What does the unsupported expression of emotions under mental and emotional stress do to us? Response to stress is a function of the autonomic nervous system that has two components: sympathetic and parasympathetic. The sympathetic nervous system "sympathizes with us" and produces the stress hormone cortisol which we need to "survive" the stressor. The parasympathetic system controls the "relaxation response" designed to bring the body back to equilibrium. So, prolonged expressive response to stressors produces an imbalance in the activities of the sympathetic and parasympathetic nervous system; at the end, the system is left in a permanent state of sympathetic arousal.

In this way, chronic irritability and nervous tension can lead to sleeplessness. And chronic irritability combined with competitiveness and domination—both instinctual negative emotions—gives rise to downright hostility. Eventually, what was previously mental hyperactivity expressed through conditioned programs of the brain becomes manifest in the physical organs, which all begin to function at an increased level, producing disease of the involved organs. Often, the disease settles down in one organ only.

If the expressiveness of the emotional response settles down in the circulatory system, we get heart disease, hypertension, etc. If the expression occurs through the gastrointestinal digestive system, the result is ulcer. If the expression occurs through the elimination systems of the body, the diseases are irritable bowel syndrome, bladder disorders, etc. If the expression takes place through the immune system, causing excess immune reaction to antigens, the result is allergy. If the expression is through the respiratory system, the disease is asthma.

Why does the expression settle down in one organ as opposed to another? This has been the million-dollar, unsettled question in traditional medicine. In quantum science, this has to do with the response of the vital software V-organ, where feelings originate at the chakras.

Recall that different types of emotion are felt at different chakras. For example, irritability and anger are felt at the navel chakra when our desires are thwarted. The quick processing of meaning as hyperactive people do, amplifies the feeling at that chakra. In this way, chronic irritability will express itself in the organs of the navel chakra, most often as peptic ulcer.

Hostility means looking at the world as enemy, as not-me. When irritability gives way to hostility, as when combined with competitiveness and tendency to dominate others, the immune system overreacts, causing inflammation of the heart chakra organs.

If you direct the hostile reaction at people in intimate relationship with you, you will become abusive in those heated moments. But of course just because you are abusive in those moments, you don't quit on love, so your immune system function is not affected; but eventually, the organ affected is the heart. Heart disease will result.

Let's spell out the details of how coronary blockage—a major source of disease and death—takes place. The immune system produces inflammation in the arteries. If additionally, vata-kapha doshas exist, cholesterol can accumulate due to kapha dosha; vayu is not available to clean up the arteries due to vata dosha, the result is blockage. If this happens in the coronary arteries, the blockage can be fatal.

If the hostile reaction is directed toward the environment and people around you because you don't have an intimate relationship, then you are a quitter of love, and the organ affected is the immune system itself.

Immune system malfunction will lead to cancer in a similar scenario as above. Abnormal cells accumulate due to aggravated kapha; aggravated vata prevents clearance of the accumulated abnormality, eventually becoming cancer when additionally the immune system malfunctions. In this way, emotionally expressive people of so-called type-A personality are found to be prone to both heart disease and cancer.

Hostility is not the only problem with irritability and competitiveness. Advanced stages of irritability and competitiveness can also give rise to frustration, which is a throat chakra feeling (arising when the throat chakra is depleted of vital energy). When the mind gets into the action due to the dosha of hyperactivity, the feeling of frustration is amplified. Repeated amplification of frustration expresses itself as a throat chakra disease, e.g. asthma if there is already a kapha-vata joint aggravation.

If the emotion expressed is fear and insecurity, the chakra involved is the root chakra. When amplified by the mind, this may lead to diseases of the root chakra organs, such as serious constipation and irritable bowel syndrome.

When the feeling involves the sex chakra, as in the feeling of unfulfilled lust, mental amplification gives rise to diseases of the sex chakra, causing malfunction of the pathway to the bladder. The enlargement of the bladder, responsible for urinary problems such as waking up frequently at night to urinate for many males of age sixty and above, is a disease of this kind.

I (Amit) had a friend in his sixties who used to keep naked pictures of *Playboy* models on his desk with the sign that said, "Dirty old men need love too." He was right. Love is a preventive remedy of all organ-expressions of immune system malfunction.

SUPPRESSION OF EMOTIONS

When consciousness suppresses an emotion through the intermediary of the brain and its connection to the physical organs through nerves and neuropeptides, the vital body movements in the corresponding chakra are suppressed, affecting the physiological functions of the physical organs there. This is what is responsible for the somatic effect, the experience of illness at a specific organ site in response to a stressor. In particular, if the emotion of love is suppressed, the immune system malfunctions. We may get cancer.

Immune system malfunction is also responsible for autoimmune diseases such as arthritis at a knee joint, but it is more complicated than just that. The way the immune system recognizes the cells of an organ in the body as "me" is to leave a marker at the organ during early development. However, if the organ physically changes due to wear and tear as a knee joint, then the marker becomes useless, the malfunctioning immune system cannot recognize the cells of the organ as the body's own and attacks them.

Suppression at the brow chakra may be responsible for tension headaches and migraines, even depression. And suppression at the crown chakra leads to peculiar diseases connected with the parietal lobe and physical body images.

Some teenage girls are found to be body-conscious to the extreme (this is further exacerbated by the current culture of Instagram), so much so that they even tend to starve themselves to death—the disease of anorexia.

How does bio-energetics work? The suppression-repression dynamic is most commonly memorized in the muscles because when we are defensive, we tend to tense our muscles. As we repress the mental-emotional experience, we also repress the muscle tension and they never fully relax. In this way, a muscle makes a memory of the suppressed emotion, a memory when the muscle is fixated in a certain position and cannot relax that position. In this way, repression of the mind translates as the repression of muscular activity. The muscles retain a "body memory," so to speak, of the emotional trauma suppressed.

What does repeated suppression of an emotional response mean, then, in terms of muscular tension memory? Quantum physics says this:

in subsequent experiences of that stimulus, just as the consciousness is not allowed to collapse certain mental states of awareness of the emotional response, the particular muscle memory is not collapsed either. So this particular muscle is not reactivated by subsequent emotional experiences because the mental defense mechanism is always aroused.

Such suppressed emotions all over the body gives rise to serious diseases such as fibromyalgia—a state of widespread muscle pain. A related disease is chronic fatigue syndrome, for which the main physical body symptom is total fatigue. If feelings are suppressed in all the body chakras, practically all the corresponding vital body movements will be suppressed. This may manifest as a general lack of vitality explaining chronic fatigue. If the feeling suppression involves more the structural parts of the body in which the organs are embedded, but not the organs themselves, the lack of vital energy may be felt as pain all over the body: fibromyalgia.

A comment: Pain is interesting because being a feeling it must have a vital energy connection. And yet, the role of the nerves is also undeniable, since by numbing them (local anesthesia), we can numb pain also. So, pain is a mentalized feeling, a feeling connected with the suppression of the movement of vital energy at any structural part of the body and interpreted by the mind as pain, because it is unpleasant. This is a very persistent mentalization, obviously millions of years old, and has much survival value.

DISEASE-PRONE PERSONALITY

Is there such a thing as a personality type that develops a specific mind-body disease? For example, coronary heart disease is connected with type-A personality, people who react quickly with anger and hostility, especially hostility, to a stress-producing situation. Is such connection valid for other kinds of disease in which the mind may be involved?

At one point, there was a considerable amount of literature

connecting cancer exclusively to type-B personality associated with emotion suppression and non-assertiveness, even hopelessness. But cancer can result also for the Type-A personality, negating this conclusion.

In truth, there is clinical support only for the idea that there is such a thing as a disease-prone personality. Howard S. Freidman and Stephanie Booth-Kewley were motivated to study the specific connection of personality types for asthma, coronary heart disease, ulcers, headaches, and arthritis. They found little evidence of any specific connection of any of the above-mentioned diseases to a personality type. Instead, their data showed the existence of a disease-prone personality involving depression, anger/hostility, anxiety, etc.

This finding is entirely consistent with the idea of mind/brain dosha. Some people have a mixture of mind-brain doshas which manifests as personalities with more than one predominant disposition toward emotion: both suppression of emotion (depression) and expression (irritability, hostility, etc.). All we can say about such people is that they are disease prone.

Q&A

If I have a disease-prone personality, doesn't it seem that I am responsible for my disease? Should I then feel guilty?
Authors: This is a good question. Many New Age teachers will squarely put the blame on your shoulders for your ailments—"Why are you hiding behind your heart disease?"—but in truth, do we really know that your disease has been produced at the mind level and not at the vital or the physical level? And even if it is at the mind level, it is the conditioned ego that is responsible when you are a little helpless. The fact is, we don't usually know, we cannot know without the power of deep intuition.

At the same time, what prevents you from taking responsibility for healing yourself if you do want to be healed? When you take such responsibility, then only you can truly engage with the techniques of mind-body healing that depend not only on your body's wisdom but also on your creativity.

THE LEGENDARY DR. HAMER

According to the German physican Dr. Ryke Geerd Hamer (1935-2017), no real diseases exist; rather, what established medicine calls a "disease" is actually a "special meaningful program of nature" (*sinnvolles biologisches Sonderprogramm*) to which bacteria, viruses, and fungi belong in response to your emotional conflicts. Hamer's theory of medicine claims to explain every disease and treatment according to those premises, and to thereby obviate traditional medicine. The cure is always the resolving of the conflict. Some treatments, like *chemotherapy* or pain-relieving drugs like morphine, are deadly according to Hamer.

Dr. Hamer was studying the testicular cancer of his son. Dr. Hamer then noted that on brain CT scans every testicular and ovarian cancer patient had a dark spot in the brain. He concluded that not only cancer but all disease is triggered by unexpected shocks and traumas affecting the brain. Later, he came to the conclusion that various related smaller emotional triggers can accumulate over years or even decades to manifest as disease.

Dr. Hamer summarized his postdoctoral research at Germany's Tübingen University in October 1981: "I searched for cancer in the cell and I have found it in the form of a wrong coding in the brain."

Dr. Hamer was the first who could provide scientific evidence that diseases do not originate in an organ/tissue as previously assumed but in the brain as a result of unexpected conflict shocks. The result of his research is a detailed scientific chart (a brain map) that indicates from exactly what area in the brain a specific disease is controlled and to what specific type of conflict the physical symptom is biologically related. Dr. Hamer's method of brain scan analysis offers a most reliable tool for both diagnosis and prognosis, and does not indicate that "Hamer desperately needed to get his position back in the medical society," wrote Caroline Markolin, a German literature Ph.D. who later became an exponent of Hamer's New Medicine. Could there be such programs in our brain? If so, what produces them?

UNNECESSARY MENTALIZATION OF FEELINGS CAN BE HARMFUL TO OUR HEALTH

A feeling is a feeling is a feeling. It is neither inherently good nor bad. The value we give to feelings, and our likes and dislikes, are created through the mind's "job" of giving meaning to everything it is able to process. This is one way we mentalize our value-neutral feelings.

American anthropologists have found that some Eskimo natives they encountered did not have a word for anger. This must mean that anger, as an emotive expression, was traditionally not a part of the social world of these Eskimos. Of course, this changed after their interaction with the anthropologists began: They had to coin a word for anger to describe the irritability and frustrations for describing the behavior of the anthropologists.

Consider a feeling like fear. If a tiger comes into my immediate environment, fear, the rush of vital energy out of my root and navel chakras, gives me the physical adrenaline rush that helps my "flight" or (rarely, in this case) "fight" response. It is a feeling that is necessary for the survival of our species, and no doubt evolution has helped to make it an instinct. But what if you fantasize about a tiger in your living room who is really your boss and you become afraid as a result of your fantasy? You will get a shiver through your body (fear) and butterflies in your stomach (anxiety) because of your fantasy, and an adrenaline rush (stress response) as well, but it is all a case of mind over vital body, an unnecessary mentalization of an otherwise useful natural feeling. Note also that even the mentally lazy cannot avoid health hazards due to fantasy emotions.

chapter eleven

QUANTUM SCIENCE OF THE HEART CHAKRA AND WOMEN'S BREAST CANCER

Having covered the theory of chronic disease as mind-body disease, in this chapter we will discuss some specific cases of this phenomenon. I (Amit) had major lifestyle issues before turning seriously to soul-making. I have suffered through irritable bowel syndrome, stomach ulcer, and coronary heart disease. I am now past eighty and Alzheimer's is a real threat. However, breast cancer is the disease which played a crucial role in my discovery of the science of the heart, so that is where I will begin.

THE SCIENCE OF THE HEART, LOVE, AND CANCER

The feeling of love is associated with the heart chakra. Can we feel with the heart chakra as we think with the neocortex, as a self that experiences a feeling separate from itself? Just as we experience a thought separate from the "I" who is our consciousness that has identified itself with the brain, is there a self that is associated with the heart chakra? The answer lies in Antoine de Saint-Exupéry's evocative novella *The Little Prince*:

It is only with the heart that one can see rightly; what is essential is invisible to the eye [and the brain].

The answer is, yes, the heart does have a self, and there is new evidence from neuroscience supporting this idea.

I (Amit) have been studying consciousness experientially through many spiritual practices—some traditional, some original—and intellectually through quantum physics for over forty years. Eventually, my exploration led to the discovery of a science for the heart's self-identity.

Love and heart talk has much to do with one of the most dreadful diseases of modern times: cancer, which is the No. 2 chronic and fatal disease today. And unlike heart disease, we have known very little about what exactly causes cancer until now.

What we did know when I began my research is that certain cells in a certain organ, let's call them rogue cells, start mutating when they divide. The first few divisions don't show much abnormality, but from the fourth division or so onward, it becomes clear that the cell somehow has gotten rid of the "cap" on its chromosome, a cap that sets a limit to how many times a cell can divide (this number is around fifty for a normal human cell). By doing experiments with human cell cultures in a test tube, the physician Leonard Hayflick discovered that human cells could divide only about fifty times, no more.

A cell without a cap is called "potentially cancerous" because it can go on dividing indefinitely. But how exactly it becomes cancerous and what causes it is shrouded in mystery.

Equally mysterious is how a cancer that starts in one organ metastasizes in another organ. It simply does, and as it does, it does not change its character. A cancerous cell that starts in the liver always remains a liver cell even when it appears in another organ.

This is easy to understand once you accept the concept of the liturgical field, which is associated with a cancerous cell that is responsible for its erratic behavior. The liturgical field is the source of the vital software that runs cellular function. Ultimately, what brings about this harmful mutation of the liturgical field is the self.

Remember, consciousness is benevolent; it goes along with your intention when you pay attention. If you don't pay attention, though, it acts on the basis of your average behavior. So if you are not paying attention, genetic predispositions and perhaps also past-life karma will determine the fate of the cells of your body. Preventive medicine, paying attention to your health, is the solution. But paying attention is easier to conceptualize than it is to put in practice in all the different contexts that life presents to us.

Naturally, we hardly know anything about how to heal cancer. Surgery, radiation treatment, or dangerous (due to side effects) chemotherapy are all procedures that often only prolong the life of a patient but reduce the quality of life, and none of the treatments can give any guarantee that the patient has been healed. The quality-of-life question stops many patients from even entering the treatment of chemotherapy.

Strictly speaking, the treatment of cancer via modern medicine, allopathy, only buys us time, but not quality time. Allopathic medicine is emergency medicine. And it would be nice to have alternatives available, especially alternatives that can truly heal and truly restore wholeness.

In the sixties, the Beatles sang, "All we need is love." But those times were immature and the hippies interpreted love very physically. Now, with the help of a new paradigm of science aborning during the last few decades that is based on quantum physics and primacy of consciousness, we know a lot more about love. We all know the saying, "Love is a many-splendored thing." But what you may not know is that one of love's many splendors is that it helps prevent certain types of cancer, maybe all cancers. Another way of saying it is this: It is downright dangerous to block the energies of love, for it may beget you cancer. On the other hand, if we cultivate the heart and proceed to explore and eventually revel in our identity with it, then cancer is unlikely.

Previously, we made a connection between love and the heart chakra, which also involved the important thymus gland, a crucial part of the immune system. Suspending the immune system momentarily enables love. Blocking the energies of love at the heart chakra produces immune system disorder. Why? Could it be that love gives the immune system a much-needed rest? Perhaps depriving the immune system of rest is like depriving the neocortex of deep sleep. The neocortex needs a rest periodically from the big job of representing manifest consciousness in the brain. Could it be the same for the immune system?

At the beginning of my research, I postulated the existence of self-identity at the heart chakra. If the block from rest is long lasting, the immune system disorder becomes so huge that the immune system is unable to kill off potentially cancerous "foreign" cells in the body anymore, leading to malignancy. This gave me a tentative theory of cancer.

The conventional medical establishment is very hard to penetrate and, unfortunately, this is no less true for the alternative medicine establishment as well, though to a lesser extent. I began to get a few invitations to speak after my book *The Quantum Doctor* was published, especially after the second edition for which Deepak Chopra wrote the foreword.

Fast-forward to 2012, when I (Amit) was invited to a conference arranged by an expert on Traditional Chinese Medicine. After I delivered my talk, the expert invited me for a private conversation. He was concerned much about the prevention of breast cancer of women, he said, and he shared some of his preliminary results. His data surprised me.

This Traditional Chinese Medicine practitioner claimed that if women pay attention to their liver and stomach and also to the meridians that connect the liver and stomach to the heart chakra, they can prevent contracting breast cancer. When Traditional Chinese Medicine practitioners say the liver, they don't literally mean the liver. They mean the vital counterpart or vital software of the liver—the V-liver. The liver meridian connects the vital counterpart of the liver with the vital counterparts of the heart chakra organs. This much I could decipher. And I was surprised too because I had thought cancer was all about caring for the immune system and letting it get proper rest, and here was the good TCM doctor talking about the liver and the stomach and the meridians.

At the time, my main interest was quantum activism—a movement to change the self and society with the principles that we learn from the quantum worldview. So, initially, I did not pay too much attention to the new data. Then another synchronicity came about. The actress Angelina Jolie was getting a double mastectomy, which was big headline news. No, she did not have breast cancer; the surgery was entirely preventive because she had been told by her oncologist that she had an 86 percent chance of contracting breast cancer because of a genetic predisposition.

The episode made me feel sad about the prejudices of the medical establishment. On the other hand, I only had admiration for Angelina Jolie, whose courage and love for her children had led her to undergo a radical mastectomy.

And frankly, the Traditional Chinese Medicine practitioner's striking results about breast cancer prevention—via paying attention to the vital counterparts of the liver and stomach and their meridians that connect to the heart chakra—were strictly empirical. No theory existed yet about why that works, so I became motivated to find a theory.

We now present this new research along with a new look at older findings. The conclusion from the research is what you have perhaps already gleaned: There is a potentiality of love that is waiting in each of us to be actualized as a self, centered around the heart chakra. Movement toward its actualization takes us to spiritual wholeness; movement away from it, if there is a lot of it, leads us to disease, including cancer, including heart disease, auto-immune disease, and even depression. The heart chakra organs—the thymus gland and the immune system, and of course the heart—are not alone in this. The liver and stomach—both naval chakra organs of self-love—are also involved in producing a strong self of the heart which not only has other love but also self-love.

In the Middle Ages, while it is true that most people lived as serfs and their material life was a struggle, it is also true that they lived within familial and socio-religious structures that tacitly recognized the importance of love for our well-being. What mind-body medicine practitioners call mental stress today is mostly the absence of love in people's lives, especially when they are old. This is the principal reason that we see the anachronism of increased life-expectancy and much decreased quality of life in people's old age. We've concluded that the most important preventative measure is that love. The quantum worldview helps you see this clearly and choose. To love or not to love is the crucial question of your wellness, especially in your old age (see Chapter 16).

Finally, a word about genetic predisposition. We now know that this means there is a high probability that some rogue cell will get rid of the cell gap that prevents cells from going on dividing indefinitely. But consciousness resorts to collapsing probabilistic behavior only when we are not paying attention and only when we are, for some reason, confused about healing intention. What this consciousness-based quantum approach suggests is that the genetic predisposition can be prevented from becoming fact by paying attention to maintaining healing intention on a regular basis.

DOES THE HEART HAVE A SELF?

When I (Amit) first developed a scientific explanation of the chakras back in the 1990s, and even when I wrote about it in *The Quantum Doctor*, I thought we should be able to experience pure feeling at all the chakras, not just the neocortex, which is the sixth chakra counting from the bottom. I thought it is just a lack of sensitivity that prevents us from these experiences. And I was prepared to give the benefit of the doubt to the female of our species. Since women have always seemed to talk a lot about feeling and heart, I thought maybe women are more sensitive than men and this is why they talk so much about the heart.

However, our experiencing self is tied up with the engagement of a tangled hierarchy that requires a cognition and memory apparatus such as the neocortex. So after some research, I concluded that there is no such tangled hierarchy within the chakras and so our visceral experience of the feeling of love has to wait until the mind gives meaning to the feeling and the tangled hierarchical quantum measurement takes place in the neocortex; only then do you experience feeling, always mixed with thought, as an emotion.

But wait: While men generally accept that their self is centered in the head, quite a few women claim that their heart "talks" to them because they know how to listen to their heart. Is this a mere metaphor for women's emotionality or is there a scientific basis for it? Could women be fooling themselves thinking that they directly experience feelings at the heart? Perhaps. However, many mystical traditions refer to the spiritual journey as a journey toward the heart. How come?

There is more than a metaphor here. First, there is the new discovery of psycho-neuro-immuno-gastro-intestinology: The brain has ongoing two-way communication with the immune system (of the heart chakra) and the gastro-intestinal system (of the navel chakra).

Second, the immune system is the second-most important body organ. Scientists are discovering that the immune system has quite a bit of autonomy.

Third, everyone knows the neocortex needs sleep every night; sleep deprivation is bad for both physical and mental health. It is easy to connect the thymus gland (of the immune system) with romantic love; romance is when the immune system function of distinguishing between me and not-me is suspended. So why do we need love? The answer must be: to give the immune system some rest. If the immune system is denied rest, immune system malfunction will occur, which can lead to many disorders such as autoimmune disease, heart disease, and cancer.

Notice that if our argumentation is correct, out of all the organs of the body, only the neocortex and the immune system seem to need regular rest. What do they have in common? The neocortex has autonomy;

it also has a tangled hierarchy and it thereby acquires a self. The immune system has autonomy, but does it also have a self and a tangled hierarchy? Let's take a look at that.

One recent surprise in neuroscience is the discovery of neurons at the heart chakra. There is no doubt that there is a cognition system at the heart chakra, as the feeling of love is an excellent way to cognize. With the bundle of nerves available, there is also the capacity to make memory. Cognition and memory—the two systems that make a tangled hierarchy—are included in the heart chakra. So, the heart chakra has a self: the heart chakra can actualize experience—pure feeling—by itself, without the brain's help.

There is a lot to emphasize about the heart. To me (Valentina), vital energy and meditative practices on the heart (such as the practices of forgiveness and gratitude) are the main way to heal, and at the same time, awaken spiritually. The journey of being and starting to manifest your human potential starts when we awaken our hearts—our spiritual hearts, of course.

More recently, neuroscientists have also discovered another little "brain," another big bundle of nerves at the navel chakra. The navel chakra has a cognition apparatus; it cognizes the feeling of self-respect or self-love. Its little brain gives it a memory apparatus. The combination makes a tangled hierarchy and manifests a self-identity centered at the navel.

In Japanese culture, the navel center is called *hara*, the self of the body; at least one spiritual culture has recognized even this center of the self for hundreds of years. To be fair, even in our modern culture, creative people do talk about "gut feelings" that tell them about the veracity of an intuitive experience.

The important question is why do we not hear the small voice of the heart and the small voice of the navel chakra, these pure feelings associated with the actualization of experience at these chakras? We think this has to do with evolution and culture and is perhaps the main contributing factor for the male-female difference.

In this way, if there is no love in one's life, immune system function is never suspended, and prolonged occurrence of this may produce immune system disorders. For a woman, certain situations such as bereavement can lead to a prolonged suspension of love in her life and thus immune system malfunctioning. This then can produce breast cancer.

The identification of the absence of love as the source of immune system malfunctioning gives us an extra handle in our effort to understand cancer. It brings to the fore the role of the mind in causing vital energy blocks. To starve the heart chakra of love—unless fulfilment is achieved with only the desired partner, and nobody else—is often a mental decision that suppresses the feeling of love toward others. Thus, certain types of cancer, breast cancer in particular, can be recognized as a mind-body disease.

Again, from the perspective of mind-body disease, prevention is the best policy to deal with the problem. Historically, people were encouraged to grieve more than they naturally would. Family support made up for some of the missing romantic love. Now, with family connections weakened, with a cancer-prone environment, and an exponential increase in emotional stress, we should do the opposite and discourage prolonged mourning.

This idea can be tested. Just do a clinical study to see if it is true that grieving women show greater incidents of breast cancer.

NEW DIAGNOSTIC AVENUES

Breast cancer that is caused by vital energy blocks at the heart chakra can be diagnosed with a quite simple noninvasive procedure. For a while, Kirlian photography, images of the skin made through contact photography and high-voltage electricity, have been found to convey information about our emotional states. Kirlian photography works because biophysicists have discovered that besides the biochemical body, we have an electromagnetic body at the skin. Like all organs, the skin, too, has a vital correlate whose movements are connected to the vital movements of the correlates of organs inside the body. In this way, a Kirlian electrical photograph at the skin in the area of the heart chakra can tell us about the vital energy block of that chakra.

Reportedly, physicians in India are already detecting very early cancer through this technique, with their results later verified by biopsy, and steps to healing have been taken with immensely improved success rates of eliminating the cancer.

In particular, I have heard reports that a Dr. Chauhan in India has looked for and found evidence of vital energy blocks in many grieving women via measurements with Kirlian photography. He has then tested these women with biopsies and in many cases has been able to intervene early and save the women from having to undergo mastectomy.

THE FINAL PIECE OF THE PUZZLE

There is still one more puzzle: Love occurs when the immune system is momentarily suspended, when we stop defending ourselves and become vulnerable to a (potential) partner. But any experience requires the collapse or actualization of new potentiality for the software of some organ. The heart is not just a blood pump.

Clarity on this subject came to me (Amit) when one day Valentina drew my attention to the previously cited Heart Math Data. When we love, the heart's movements become more coherent as shown by EKG measurements. Coherence is a sure-fire sign of quantum behavior. Bingo! It is the heart, after all, which is elevated to a new function: love. The heart is where the self is: at the heart chakra.

CONNECTING EVERYTHING: A COMPLETE THEORY OF HOW TO PREVENT BREAST CANCER

Now let's look at the breakthrough that this new data and quantum science gives us. Not only does the heart have a self, but so does the navel chakra. Add to that the male-female dichotomy: males have a strong navel but a weak heart; females have the opposite—a strong heart but a weak navel.

A strong heart gives women the capacity for other love. Unfortunately, a weak navel means women lack the capacity of self-worth, let alone self-love. Balancing the two chakras would give the capacity for other love balanced with a capacity for self-love as well.

What the Chinese Traditional Medicine doctor and teacher Nan Lu does with his students is tantamount to balancing the heart and the navel chakra functioning. This new manner of looking at things gives us alternative ways for prevention, for example, using Tai chi, chi gong, pranayama, and many other vital energy exercises to balance the two chakras.

WHY DO CELLS GO ROGUE?

The mystery of the heart is solved, but one final mystery is still left: Why do cells in an organ go rogue, defying the Hayflick limit on cell divisions? With quantum science to guide us, an explanation can be given.

A big hint comes from studies that conclusively prove the connection of smoking to cancer of the lung and the throat. We can generalize: abuse of an organ contributes to cancer in that organ. What does abuse do? It impairs the regular functioning of the organ; disfunction of an organ translates as disconnect between the organ physiology and the vital software; the more the disfunction, the more is the disconnect.

Consciousness connects to an organ via the vital-physical connection. When the latter is compromised so is the connection of consciousness to the organ as a whole.

However, consciousness can still connect to the individual cells of the organ: cellular consciousness that looks after the interests of the cell; in other words, room is made for the cell going rogue.

chapter twelve

PREVENTIVE MEDICINE LESSON 3: HOW TO DEAL WITH MENTALIZATION

What can you do to prevent wrong mentalization in the first place? This is the subject of the next preventive lesson.

Knowing that faulty meaning contributes to our illnesses and diseases, if you fall sick, you may even be tempted to contemplate whether the sickness could not have been caused by you and whether you are to be blamed. Alas, thinking this way will only aggravate your situation further.

If meaning is something inherent in how mind is engaged to process things, if we are helpless giving disease-causing meaning to our experiences in the world including the diseases we suffer through, what is our best strategy in dealing with the mind? Some people believe that thinking of disease objectively is the best from this point of view alone. But as the physician Larry Dossey, in his book *Meaning and Medicine*, correctly points out, denying meaning also means assigning negative meaning.

Denying the meaning of our illnesses is like atheists denying the existence of God—they become more obsessed than necessary. If only we could be truly agnostic.

So what is a good strategy? As Epictetus said, "Things in themselves are always neutral; it is our perception which makes them appear positive or negative." If we apply a negative mental meaning to an event, it causes an incongruence with our normal state of happiness. Instead, suppose we interpret everything so that congruence is maintained?

The East Indian mystic Swami Sivananda gave a wonderful overall strategy to deal with the meaning giver mind, which we will share with you.

A king had a ministerial companion whom he liked very much except for one thing that irritated him to no end. The minister had the habit of saying, "Whatever happens is for the good," to whatever happened around him, good or bad. So one day, the king cut his thumb while fiddling around with a knife, and the minister who was there promptly said, "Everything that happens is for the good." This comment made the king very angry and he threw the minister into the jail. To console himself, he went hunting in the forest, alone.

Lo and behold, he must have gone quite a distance and beyond his kingdom because he came across a tribe of people who took him captive. Unfortunately for the king, this was a tribe that sacrificed human beings to their deity. So the king was taken to a tribe's priest to be offered as a human sacrifice. But the priest, while bathing the king in preparation for him to be killed, discovered his cut thumb. Since a defective person could not be offered to the deity, he rejected the king, who was then released.

On his way back to the palace, the king thought long and hard about what had happened and realized that the minister's saying was correct; the cut thumb had actually saved his life. So, as soon as he was back, he released his minister and told him, "You were right about me; everything that happened to me was for my good after all. But I threw you in the dungeon for what you said, which did not seem to do you any good. How do you explain that?"

The minister replied, "Oh, great king. Your throwing me into jail saved also my life. Otherwise, I'd have accompanied you to hunting, been taken captive, and since I do not have any blemishes, I would have been offered as the human sacrifice."

New Age types will find an easy recipe for emotional intelligence in this story, but the question is, how did the minister develop this attitude? The answer is most revealing. It is certainly not easy.

MEDITATION: THIS TOO SHALL PASS

You do not have much control as a child about how you grow up. So there will always be people of various brain doshas unless we drastically change society as a whole, particularly in the area of parenting and education.

You can, as a grownup, make lifestyle changes. Is there an alternative way to handle your emotions other than suppression and expression and the superficial New Age advice, "Intend that all is okay and negativity will go away." Yes, there is: meditation.

Negative emotions are automatic responses involving the amygdala and bypassing the neocortex. Meditation slows down the psyche and the brain organs, which is one of meditation's major virtues. It buys us time to watch the response, as the neocortex comes into play, to the stimulus arising as we act.

Of course, the negative emotional response is fast and unconscious. So we also need some positive emotional brain circuits to come into play. We need these to cultivate via transformation practices such as giving, forgiving, etc. In this way, we gradually, with practice, can realize that the response, suppression, or expression, passes; we don't have to be stuck on the conditioned response and activate the motor organs of the brain. In other words, we can engage our freedom to say no to continuing in the state of conditioned choices for action. In time, we can build so many brain circuits involving the hippocampus and bypassing the amygdala—so many positive emotional brain circuits in an area of the brain called Anterior Cingulate Cortex (ACC)—using the creative process and make them available without effort, that the amygdala's circuits are basically neutralized. This makes the process of returning to equilibrium after an emotional upset even faster.

This way of dealing with stressors can eliminate a major source of your unhappiness in today's individualistic society, and thus hugely contribute to your overall health and happiness.

Can we learn not to mentalize emotions? Slowing down the mind enables us to examine more clearly how we give meaning to a particular feeling and realize after some practice that we do not have to give the conditioned meaning to a stressor. We do not have to fear the boss the way we need to fear a tiger.

Also generally, there are more stressors in our lives because of the materialist style of living in high standards, having to have jobs that do not satisfy us. You have come in this incarnation in an economically advanced society that requires a lot of rajas. This shows that you are an "old" soul. You most likely have a dharma—a preferred archetype—that you chose to explore in this life. But the sociocultural environment prevents you from following your dharma. If this rings true, try to become aware of your dharma. And if you find your dharma—the archetype of your choice, try to follow it; that will bring you happiness.

Even if all this effort of seriously exploring an archetype does not fit with your lifestyle, do consider the issue of congruence: synchronizing your life with how you make your livelihood.

MORE ABOUT AVOIDING MENTALIZATION

The mind naturally turns to dominate the vital domain of our experience by giving meaning to meaning-neutral feelings—mentalization. The trick is to change this habit pattern, so that mind can turn toward the supramental instead, where it is the servant.

So we observe the ways we mentalize our feelings, our specific pattern for giving meaning to our feelings. Once we know our pattern, with utter honesty, we become open to change. And remember, changing a pattern is always done best by taking a creative quantum leap.

A creative quantum leap of the mind always means a shift in the context with which we process meaning. Our contexts become so fixated because reason works best within a fixed set of beliefs—a belief system. If even one of these beliefs changes, the whole system may have to be questioned. And the conditioned ego-mind hates that, fears that.

The mistake we make is to think that we can change our perception of meaning just by reading something, or following a teacher, or even engaging in practice, but that is just preparation.

Have you ever been to a Zen master's teaching? He may pick up a hand fan and ask you, "What is it?" If you say, "It is a fan," he will say, "I will hit you," suggesting, if you are subtle enough to comprehend it, that a fan can also be used as something to hit with.

But here's the thing: If you wise up and say, "It is something to hit with," the Zen Master still won't be satisfied. He may say something like, "Thirty percent," at best.

So what's going on? In his famous book on Zen, *The Three Pillars of Zen*, the author Roshi Philip Kapleau describes the state to which he leapt after a five-day zendo. He ran to his teacher, took the fan from him and hit him with it. He then scratched his own body with it and used the fan as a scale. All these shenanigans of joyful spontaneity left no doubt in his teacher that the student was acting from his quantum self, a state in which our action comes from certainty, not cleverness.

You cannot choose health just by wishing it, which is cleverness. When you choose health from the spirit of exploration, life style change starts taking place. After a creative quantum leap, we gain a sense of direction that further helps. When we make a quantum leap of fundamental creativity, we have certainty in our pursuit; then only you are able to master the energy to make lifestyle changes as you know necessary. But you know what; it is all a journey in happiness, in well-being.

PART THREE

UNLEASHING the FULL POWER of QUANTUM INTEGRATIVE MEDICINE

chapter thirteen

PREVENTIVE MEDICINE LESSON 4: NUTRITION

This chapter will look at how to nourish the five bodies of the human being via a process we call quantum yoga. Yoga, in this context, means integration. Our various bodies are not independent of one another; hence proper nutrition for healthy preventive maintenance needs yoga. Since we are using quantum principle, quantum yoga.

We begin with the physical level. But first, do a simple exercise: develop awareness of the various states you experience during a typical day

1. Try to remember what happened during the day. In which physical, emotional, mental state did you start your day?
2. What states did you experience during the day?
3. In what kind of state of spirit are you now?
4. Was there an energetical/thinking pattern that was repeating within you?

THE PHYSICAL-VITAL LEVEL

Food is a vital part of our physical nourishment, but in recent years we have received a lot of conflicting information about what to eat and what not to eat. As a result, many of us have lost touch with our natural body signals; we have become busy with focusing on the outside, without listening to what our bodies are asking for that we need from the inside. The nutritional recommendations given here are not rules for you to adhere to. This journey is not about "you must eat this and not eat that"—rather, it is about listening to all your five bodies for what it needs to feel nourished and then engaging appropriately.

Food is for both nutrition and pleasure. Our cells need food to maintain and multiply themselves, our organs need nutrition to function optimally, so fresh, natural foods with good vital energy are recommended. However, our brains do have pleasure circuits and if non-harmful but not optimal foods serve that purpose, we should indeed occasionally indulge. The challenge is to keep this occasional dalliance as harmless as possible.

Certain energetic conditions, such as giving thanks or saying a prayer before eating, also raises the nutrition we get from the vital energy of food. It is also worth noting that vegetarian food has a higher vital energy (moreover, it is relatively undifferentiated) than non-vegetarian food and fresh unprocessed vegetarian meals digest more easily too. When we, the authors, teach in India, we eat three high-carb, satisfying vegetarian meals a day with very little snacking in between, and yet neither of us nor anyone else on the team (mostly Westerners) gains weight. The reason? It is because we make sure that we are satisfied on every level. The meal itself is fresh and balanced, incorporating all six tastes as much as practicable as recommended by Ayurveda: sweet, sour, pungent, astringent, bitter, and salty. Given that we have an inbuilt mechanism to seek pleasure, this combination of food when adjusted for personal emphasis on tastes according to your dosha-prakriti is perfect for providing the pleasure factor.

We must remember that when we ingest meats, not only are we ingesting all the chemicals that the animal was given prior to being slaughtered, but we are also ingesting the fear that the animal endured before and during the slaughter-process. (Even after death, which is brain death, the tissues we eat still retain their non-local integrity that include their correlation with the vital.)

We also need to keep the pleasure factor in mind when we think about how much to eat. We're all born with the ability to sense hunger and fullness, but many of us lose touch with these natural signals because we're influenced by both external and emotional factors. Additionally, processed foods can affect our ability to experience satiety too. We recommend that you practice tuning in to your body's hunger and fullness signals. Consider the following points.

- Learn what real hunger feels like. The onset of hunger is gradual, remember that. Don't eat according to your ritual if you are not hungry.
- How often do you snack, and are you hungry when you snack?
- Are you someone that never feels hungry? This can happen if our eating patterns are erratic and if we eat unhealthy processed foods. One of the simplest ways to overcome this is to establish an eating routine based on hunger, focus on ingesting fresh, unprocessed foods, and eliminate snacking as much as practicable.

Getting in tune with your fullness signal also may take some practice. Here are some things to consider.

It takes time for our brain to register that we have eaten as needed, so chewing thoroughly, eating slowly and tuning in every now and then to your satisfaction level during your meal is a good idea.

There is a difference between being comfortably full and when you feel full. Many people equate adequate eating with the feeling of being full, but in truth you have already overeaten. When you're comfortably full, you should feel satisfied on every level but not uncomfortable in any way. Sleepiness after a meal is a sign that you may have eaten too much.

The most important sign that you have not overeaten is the feeling of expansiveness that should follow every meal that nourishes you. Look for it every time you eat. This is when pleasure gives way to happiness.

FASTING

> *"Everyone has a physician inside him or her; we just have to help it in its work. The natural healing force [intention] within each one of us is the greatest force in getting well. Our food should be our medicine. Our medicine should be our food. But to eat when you are sick is to feed your sickness."* —Hippocrates

Fasting has not received as much attention as it should when it comes to the world of health and medicine. That's because you can't really make any money off it. The pharmaceutical science studies used in medical schools to teach doctors about human health simply don't focus enough on fasting for doctors to be knowledgeable in the subject. Doctors also learn very little about nutrition and are trained to prescribe drugs as a result.

I (Valentina) am very fond of periodic fasting (especially during the equinoxes and solstices). I prefer water fasting. And I have seen fasting's positive effect on multiple levels, health-wise. We even have a fasting group, and it is so much easier to fast when you do it in a group. The body has its great wisdom, we just need to give it a break, once in a while. The same do-be-do-be-do principle at work. The digestive system needs a regular break, which has the effect of bringing up that natural "fire" of the body, by awakening the quantum, and that will simply allow Health to elevate to a higher physiological level.

Even a negative emotional state can be "cleansed" through fasting. Simply pay attention and notice all the processes that take place in your being. The way you start and end a fasting is important, and also what you do, especially your attitude in between. There are clinics in the world (in Russia, for example) where, under medical supervision and laboratory testing, patients heal from some of the worst diseases, through fasting. Usually, these clinics are built in the woods or in the middle of nature. People fast and meet for yoga, Tai chi sessions, walks in nature, dancing, and other natural therapies.

Dr. Jason Fung, a Toronto-based nephrologist, is one of a growing number of scientists and doctors to create awareness about the tremendous health benefits that can be achieved from fasting. It's one of the oldest dietary interventions in the world and has been practiced for thousands of years. If proper fasting was bad or harmful in any way, as some doctors suggest, it would have been known by now, and studies would not be emerging now showing the health benefits that can be achieved from fasting regularly. A study published in the journal *Cell* shows how a fasting diet can trigger the pancreas to regenerate itself, which works to control blood sugar levels and reverse symptoms of diabetes. This verifies the quantum science prediction that when the digestive navel organs (the stomach, etc.) temporarily suspend their function, the pancreas makes a quantum leap to more healthy function that generates the feeling of self-worth. Besides such quantum leaps should help heal Type-II diabetes.

Mark Mattson, one of the foremost researchers of the cellular and molecular mechanisms underlying multiple neurodegenerative disorders like Parkinson's and Alzheimer's diseases, has shown through his work that fasting can have a tremendous effect on the brain, and could prevent or even reverse the symptoms of multiple neurodegenerative disorders.

Other studies have shown how fasting actually fights cancer and triggers stem cell regeneration. There is absolutely no evidence, for the average person, that fasting can be dangerous. If you're on prescription medication, or experience other medical problems, then there are obviously exceptions. But it's quite clear that the human body was designed to go long periods of time without food, and that it's completely natural.

> "Why is it that the normal diet is three meals a day plus snacks? It isn't that it's the healthiest eating pattern, now that's my opinion but I think there is a lot of evidence to support that. There are a lot of pressures to have that eating pattern, there's a lot of money involved. The food industry—are they going to make money from skipping breakfast like I did

today? No, they're going to lose money. If people fast, the food industry loses money. What about the pharmaceutical industries? What if people do some intermittent fasting, exercise periodically and are very healthy, is the pharmaceutical industry going to make any money on healthy people?"
—Dr. Mark Mattson, *The Intermittent Fasting Revolution*

Dr. Jason Fung, with Jimmy Moore, cowrote the book *The Complete Guide to Fasting: Heal Your Body Through Intermittent, Alternate-Day, and Extended Fasting*. It's a great book that puts to rest the fears and myths associated with extended water fasting. (Dr. Fung has also published *The Obesity Code: Unlocking the Secrets of Weight Loss*.)

RECOMMENDATION FOR BEGINNERS

"Humans live on one-quarter of what they eat; on the other three-quarters live their doctor." —Egyptian pyramid inscription

One recommended way of dieting, which was tested by the BBC's Michael Mosley in order to reverse his diabetes, high cholesterol, and other problems associated with his obesity, is known as the 5:2 Diet. On the 5:2 plan, you cut your food down to one-fourth of your normal daily calories for two fasting days (about 600 calories for men and about 500 for women), while consuming plenty of water and tea. On the other five days of the week, you can eat normally.

Another way to do it is to restrict your food intake between the hours of 12:00 p.m. and 8:00 p.m. daily, while not eating during the hours outside of that time. This 16:8 diet is getting some traction nowadays. I (Amit) myself use it not just for dieting but as a regular eating ritual.

Fasting is sparking the interest of many because, along with this consciousness shift, comes awareness of a world beyond our physical one. This realm deals with near-death experiences, quantum physics, parapsychology, our overall spiritual nature, and the proof that's emerging that we are more than just this body, and that human beings do indeed have a spiritual nature.

The fact that modern science, in many instances, is catching up to ancient wisdom is quite exciting. This is happening not only in neuroscience and quantum physics, but in healthcare as well.

Yoshinori Ohsumi, a Japanese cell biologist, was awarded the Nobel Prize in Physiology or Medicine for his discoveries on how cells recycle their content, a process known as *autophagy*, a Greek term for "self-eating." It is a crucial process to try to understand. During starvation, cells break down proteins and nonessential components and reuse them for energy. Cells also use autophagy to destroy invading viruses and bacteria, sending them off for recycling, and to get rid of damaged structures. The process is thought to go awry in cancer, infectious diseases, immunological diseases and neurodegenerative disorders. Disruptions in autophagy are also thought to play a role in aging.

But little was known about how autophagy happens, what genes were involved, or its role in disease, and normal development until Dr. Ohsumi began studying the process in baker's yeast.

The process he studied is critical for cells to survive and to stay healthy. The autophagy genes and the metabolic pathways he discovered in yeast are used by higher organisms, including humans. The mutations in those genes can cause disease. His work led to a new field and inspired hundreds of researchers around the world to study the process and opened a new area of inquiry.

There are five crucial ways to activate your autophagy: eat a high-fat, low-carb diet; limit protein intake to 15 grams per day; once a week, practice intermittent fasting; exercise regularly; and get restorative sleep.

CARING FOR THE VITAL BODY

Balancing the vital body between creativity and conditioning—yin and yang—is extremely important for well-being. We have already mentioned previously that traumatic suppression of vital energy affects the physical body significantly, and both energy psychology and energy medicine are excellent modalities in order to help achieve vital energy balance.

While trauma release work may need specific guidance, there are vital energy exercises that we can all do that will help to rebalance our energies. We have provided a few exercises below.

SACRED MEDITATION

Start off by rubbing your palms together and then bring them apart about half an inch (rather like the *namaste* style of greeting.) You will be able to feel a tingling sensation in the hands, which is the movement of prana (vital energy) in the skin. Now, outstretch your arms so that your palms are facing the sky, and invite all of the healing energy that the universe (all the biota of the universe, that is) is sending you. This will energize your palms further, and you are now ready to give a friend some pranic healing.

Ask the friend to lie down in a comfortable position and to remain receptive to the process. Now bring your energized palms close to each of your friend's major chakras with the intention of healing for a minute or so. Start with the crown chakra and move across all the chakras in turn (crown, third-eye, throat, heart, navel, sex, and root). Please note, no physical touch is required.

PRANAYAMA: BREATHING DEEPLY WITH AWARENESS

Special emphasis must be given to breathing practices called pranayama in chakra-cleansing practices. Breathing practices are also essential for chakra balancing. Many of us take shallow breaths, where we feel the breath predominantly in our throat and nose, but when we focus on breathing deeply, we draw breath into the stomach. One such exercise is simply breathing deeply with awareness. For this exercise sit comfortably and draw slow, focused, relaxed breaths into the stomach, holding each breath for a few seconds while observing what is happening in your body, and then exhale.

The movement of prana in the vital body parallels the movement of air as we breathe oxygen into the organs along the spine; this is the basis of pranayama. The object of pranayama is to control the movement of prana between chakras; clearly, when one arrives at such control, then the chakras can easily be balanced and maintained in that state.

As we slow our breathing down, we also slow down the movement of prana along the nadis (energy-carrying channels). The nadis are connected to the chakras, and hence slowing our breathing down also helps to slow the organs at the chakras as well. This will result not only in an increased awareness of pranic movement but also allow unconscious processing and enable us to collapse new movements of prana and will even improve the chance of experiencing creative quantum leaps.

ALTERNATE NOSTRIL BREATHING

This is a great exercise for activating the parasympathetic nervous system, which helps with relaxation and regeneration. It also helps to balance the body's energy systems. It also obviously helps balance an overactive sympathetic nervous system when one is under stress.

Make sure that you are sitting comfortably; relax and focus on normal breathing. You will be using your right hand, specifically your thumb and ring finger, for this exercise. Gently close your right nostril with your thumb, and exhale slowly through your left nostril. Next, use your ring finger to close your left nostril, and then gently exhale through your right nostril. Keeping your left nostril closed, inhale through your right nostril. Now, close your right nostril with your thumb again and exhale through your left nostril. This is one cycle. Repeat this five times and then return to normal breathing.

KAPALAVATI, OR "RADIANT FOREHEAD"

Sit comfortably and start by taking in a small inhalation, and then practice forced exhalation of breath, using only your stomach muscles. Practice this between 20 and 40 times a minute. When this exercise is done properly (you may need a teacher for this), you will experience a few moments of breathlessness when you stop. Take your time to return to normal breathing. Notice that when you are without breath, you are also without thought. This thoughtless state makes way for quantum-self experiences and you may find a heightened sense of intuition.

There are also other simple practices that you can do which will help to balance the energy at the chakras. For example, walking barefoot on soil or grass is very good for the root chakra. Laughing meditation, which is the practice of laughing without stopping is very good for the navel and the heart chakra. For the throat chakra, free expression of creativity, such as singing, even if it's just in the shower, or chanting will help to balance this area.

Alternating a focused repetition of a mantra (concentration meditation) and the relaxed watching of the mind's sky (awareness meditation) helps to keep the brow chakra balanced.

GETTING TO THE PRIMORDIAL EMOTIONAL LEVEL

"Emotions are nothing bad. At their basis there are the primordial energies that can be well used. Indeed, the energy of enlightenment comes from the same source that gives birth to our daily passions and emotions."
—James Austin

Many people are sensitive to emotions but are not aware about the message in the quote above. The subtle information they receive in an emotional experience remains in the subconscious level of their minds and they don't realize it. They have a tendency to share this information in an unconscious eruptive way, because they are overwhelmed or panicked or sometimes just irritated or upset (or experiencing a mood swing) and they don't know why they do this.

Other people are aware of their sensitivity and they can identify and use the subtle information they receive from the emotional stressor. Thus, they experience less suppression and less eruptive pressure coming from their unconscious. They synchronize better their words and actions, reaching a greater success.

There are also hypersensitive people who can act efficiently, taking advantage of the accumulated information and wisdom they receive as intuition.

Most people manifest a mixture of these categories, being at times aware and other times not aware of certain aspects related to their own sensitivity, sometimes attentive upon some of them and sometimes not.

EMOTIONAL INTELLIGENCE

Intelligence is the ability to appropriately respond to a situation. For example, the intelligence that is measured by the IQ test is our problem-solving capacity, which is mental and therefore algorithmic, logical, and quantifiable.

Aside from mental intelligence, another kind of intelligence that is being touted today is emotional intelligence, thanks to popular expositions such as one by researcher Daniel Goleman called *Emotional Intelligence*. When we are faced with an emotional situation, our mental problem-solving capacity is not of much help.

So, what is emotional intelligence? The psychologist Peter Salovey defines it as capacities in five different domains of experience: knowing oneself—awareness of one's own emotional nature; emotion management; controlling and directing emotions in the service of motivation toward goals; empathy—the ability to interact with other people's emotion yet retaining one's objectivity; and finally, handling intimate relationships.

Many of the techniques of chakra medicine as well as mind-body medicine of previous chapters are designed to help us grow emotional intelligence, for example, awareness and empathy training and energy balancing between the chakras.

EXERCISES FOR EMOTIONAL AWARENESS

1. Write in your journal about three recent experiences, positive or negative, during which you recently acted upon your emotions. For example: "I asked her forgiveness because I realized how much she got hurt because of my behavior." Another example: "I saw a documentary about missing children and I was agitated all day." What physical and emotional perceptions did you have before and after the event? How did you realize what you were feeling? How the people around you react to you?
2. Describe three experiences in which other people have been emotionally sensitive or insensitive towards you. In which way has this affected you?
3. Think of a few cases when you inadvertently picked up somebody's negative emotion. Try to become more attentive to situations like this when you could be more sensitive emotionally and not pick up somebody else's negativity. Simultaneously, when such an event takes place, do your best to amplify empathy toward the person who is experiencing negativity, and use this empathic opening to find out more information about the emotionally affected person's situation and make a greater contribution to help the person. Notice what you feel after amplifying your conscious perception of the other person's emotions.

What do we notice when we keep the attention over our physical body chakra experiences? Which of the activities are we able to perceive? The easiest may be to perceive our own breathing at the stomach, or the heart activity—the heart bit. If we are able to go deeper, we may be able to gradually perceive other biochemical processes, even the vibration of our cells, and of what is called "quantum entities" that produce "inner" sound.

EXERCISE

Sit in a comfortable position with your hands palms-up on your lap. Relax and breath slowly. Focus your attention entirely upon the present moment and the inside of your body. Perceive the vital energy within your being, without which we wouldn't even live. Transfigure your body and the vital energy that is animating it.

Observe your breathing, the fresh air coming into your lungs, and the impurities being expelled; observe the succession of this cycle without interfering. Notice your heartbeat and then your pulse beat in various parts of your body. This vibration is a bit quicker than the rhythm of your breathing. Try to identify yourself with your heartbeats, without interfering in modifying the cardiac rhythm.

Scan now your entire being, your nadis, perceiving this vibration of life in your whole structure.

You can focus upon a certain organ or cellular tissue. Imagine that you are looking at the cells through a microscope and try to feel the very subtle, specific vibration, even identifying with a single cell, and perceive the immense vital force and the vibrations within the cell.

Come back gradually from the expanded state of consciousness to the ordinary state, from cell to organs and nadis, to pulse beats, to heartbeats, to breathing; become aware of a global state of regeneration within you.

In order to better understand what, how deeply, and how we feel, it is necessary to become aware of our own emotional patterns. Knowing and cultivating the healthy ones will help us make better decisions and have better relations, while knowing the negative ones will help us better understand our wounds and the energetic blockages created by these wounds. This awareness will indicate to us the aspects of emotional intelligence that we need to develop in our own being.

HOW TO BECOME AWARE OF YOUR EMOTIONAL PATTERNS

Let's travel back in time in our imagination, right to our post-birth baby period, when we were fully acting as an empathic and sensitive being centered in our feeling selves, before we developed the egoic identity and mimetic mechanisms, and before we learned to speak and created protection sheets of an interior castle. We were unitary then, like a mini sun, emitting light, love, and joy towards all those who wanted to rejoice those vibrations, coming receptively towards us. Whenever our love was reaching our parents or others near us, they were responding with the same love and empathy, validating and making our reality become even more alive. We could feel the vibration of our quantum self through a sensation that we can call *Plaisir*.

Any healthy childhood is characterized by this particular quantum self-awareness. In your imagination, bathe in this Plaisir.

On the other hand, sometimes our parents or others were manifesting fear and negativity, closing their hearts, treating us with mistrust or rejecting the spontaneous joy we were receiving from these specific vibrations of Plaisir. Maybe that is because a parent had a tough childhood and copied its patterns, convinced that all children need discipline as he or she did. Whenever our endless joy was meeting that parent's rigid, severe convictions and stony emotions, the vibration that we were perceiving was no longer soul vibration. We were feeling that something was not right but we didn't know what exactly that was, which made us feel confused and disoriented; this imprinted us with lower survival-oriented emotions, denser and darker than our own natural ones. And this is what primarily brought us the experience of a separate external world which is negative, not only separate from life and sentience, but also one to fear. All these negative perceptions perpetuated through our unconscious and separated us from our quantum self. We experienced them in the form of pain.

As a result, our beings were constantly looking for love to self-sustain. In this way, when we were children, we learned that the energy we were getting from our parents was not as unpleasant if we adapted their behavior—that is, if we imitated our parents' convictions and body postures. So, whenever we had to do it, we were copying them, renouncing ourselves to express ourselves as our parents were.

No child can manifest a natural expansiveness and creativity as long as she or he is constantly punished for this. A child gives up on expressing her love if those emotions are not reciprocated by her parents. His eyes or chest don't emanate anymore warmth if his mother's eyes remain cold, or his father's heart remains stony. The child learns to stop talking, noticing that her mother relaxes better in this way; or she learns to walk like her father to validate him, only to get his love.

Sometimes a child plays the clown, a buffoon, because funny moments make it easier to stand the long absences of his parents who are at work. The child learns to let his energy flow only in the areas where it is allowed and blocks it from other areas. He mistakes the adopting of his parents' convictions, emotional inclinations, or bodily postures with their love. If he doesn't get the validation of his quantum self, he ends up accepting what he receives from his parents in order to just survive, even if what he receives is very tiny.

These repeated abuses, these immense contractions of his being can dramatically delay a child's growth and development at all levels. And this is how many children get their first emotional habits. They learn to sit in certain postures, to manifest only certain energies, and they are seldom allowed the creative sparks of the natural light of their quantum self to shine without careful monitoring.

This is the story of many children's personality development. These children learn to define themselves in a certain way, as a certain kind of persona in certain situations, false it may be considering that he cannot function except according to certain rules.

"We cannot live the experience of our Self because our inner world is packed with past traumas. When we start eliminating this filter, the energy of light and divine love starts again to flow freely through our being," wrote Father Thomas Keating. In my (Amit's) book with Sunita

Pattani *Quantum Psychology and the Science of Happiness*, we call that filter "clouds that cover the sun (of our quantum self)."

HOW TO LET GO THE NEGATIVE EMOTIONAL PERSONALITY PATTERNS AND START FORMING POSITIVE ONES

The more unconscious we were when we adapted to our childhood to the limited external conditions, to conditioned love and partial acceptance, the more overwhelmed we may feel now, when external stimuli in the form of new stressors are incident upon us. Stimuli that do not correspond to the learnt patterns in the childhood may now seem foreign and threatening, the same as it seemed in the childhood time when we had to learn the parental patterns. They also seem to annihilate our authentic identity and block our creative emotions. And we usually first react by denying the new stressors that now confuse us so that we can hold on to our existing persona/identity.

Let's now discuss the first phase of transformation. Whenever our existing vital body gets a new stressor, it brings to the surface the suppressed blockages of childhood from the unconscious. These are associated with the first compromises that we did during childhood, with the first resignations and the first sensations of losing love. So we now have a second chance to become aware of these harmful perceptions and see them as challenges to overcome so that we transform, since we have to change anyway in order to adapting to the new challenges of new stressors.

In the second phase, we engage the *Seven Is* of the science of manifestation—*Inspiration, Intention, Intuition, Imagination, Incubation, Insight,* and *Implementation* (note that this includes the creative process)—to make the quantum leap of love to our quantum self (that we blocked during development) that now with implementation and embodiment of love in our vital software will shine within us strongly. Simultaneously, we will be able to balance the negative emotional patterns previously created. All these, of course, we cannot do overnight; it takes patience, lots of repetitions, and a great deal of self-compassion.

As we identify the emotional patterns based on fear, we will notice that some of them have at their basis the decision of running away and avoiding stress (like a phobia), while others have at the basis the decision to fight and control no matter what.

First of all, we need to start identifying what exactly does not work in our life and to understand with compassion how we got blocked in these dysfunctional patterns, to forgive ourselves and to forgive the ones who contributed to their creation, and then to identify the needed new, beneficent patterns to replace the old ones.

The next step consists of becoming fully aware of any times we manifest an unhealthy pattern and do it with a practice of a new pattern. For example, if we turned our backs on a friend for not agreeing with us, we don't need to drink vodka to calm down; rather, we can start applying a healthy pattern that includes recentering and perceiving our friend's reality so that we can understand his position better.

We don't need to indulge in self-criticizing and punishing ourselves. Rather, we say: "Oh, wow, I do the same thing: I keep isolating from people that I consider strange." Or: "I see that I keep blaming my lover because he/she is not attentive to what I want." We simply need to become aware of that pattern and become fully centered in the present moment, suspending deliberation for a moment, relaxing the mind, and then becoming aware of what we are experiencing, without modifying in any way the ambient sensation/feeling. If we feel uncomfortable, we can prolong this sensation for a few more seconds in order to become fully aware of it. In other words, we can become an observer. The purpose of this is to bring the unconscious patterns in the light of our awareness, so that we can take efficient measures.

In *Managing Anxiety*, philosopher Peter Koestenbaum said, "Anxiety is nothing but the experience of growth and maturing. If we deny it, we get sick. If we accept and fully live it, it turns into joy, safety, power, inner-centering, and character. The practical formula we should follow is this: 'Go where your pain is.'" Okay, that pain turns into joy after some creative work, and there it is, good advice to begin the process of seeing the negative as opportunity to grow.

If feelings of suppression or avoidance come, we take a break. Then we can choose again: Is there a healthy pattern that could replace the old one? For example, instead of bursting in anger because someone hurt us, we could just write down in our journal the memories from childhood when we had such an experience. Or we could let go of our tensions through yoga or Tai chi. So when we are able to let go of an unhealthy emotional pattern, we need to replace it with a healthy one. If it needs the creative process and quantum leap, so what? At the end you have something to show for your work. "You see? Now I do different."

Are you ready to go back to the state of complete openness and authenticity that you had in childhood and more? Are you ready to gain more and more participation of the quantum self in your affairs, a process we call soul-making in quantum science? Are you ready to manifest new and improved physiology in your body—new doorways of health and happiness? Do you want to be an individual in your own right? Well, this is the way to do it.

RELEASING EMOTIONAL MEMORY THROUGH THERAPY

Once we do science within the primacy of consciousness, it is easy to think in a new way about another kind of mind-body healing: psychotherapy. In psychoanalytic theory, it is assumed that people often repress the memory of a childhood trauma in their unconscious; later, unhealthy behavior arises from the processing in the unconscious. But if the subject is not aware of where his or her behavior is coming from, they cannot do anything about it. The job of psychoanalysis in mind-body healing is to make such unconscious memories conscious through therapy. More recent forms of psychoanalysis—for example, psychodynamics—is designed specifically to explore current emotional reactions (such as hostility) in terms of past memory.

Quantum science agrees with the psychoanalytic theory. Consciousness refuses to collapse traumatic memory because of the pain involved. Therapy can help to relax the fear of pain, and so when the traumatic memory surfaces in unconscious processing as a possibility, consciousness is able to recognize, remember, choose, and become aware of it. The healing power of such awareness can be enormous.

As previously mentioned, we store traumatic memory in the body in the form of unactualized states of skeletal muscle excitations. In the East Indian technique of hatha yoga, the yoga postures are designed for releasing these uncollapsed muscle tensions by becoming aware of them, then relieving pain. Such recent techniques as Rolfing, acupressure, and even touch field therapy (therapeutic tapping) are designed with the same basic idea.

Julie Motz is a nontraditional healer who works together with surgeons in hospitals (such as Stanford University Hospital). She touches a patient and his energy starts to align, vibrating in resonance with hers, and the energetic meridians that she touches raise their energy to higher chakras. She is using a healing intent, full of love, and that point of contact becomes like a magnet for beneficent vital energies that enter the patient's body through her fingers.

A form of touch therapy operating with the vital body energy involves touching certain points along meridians. Emotional freedom technique (EFT) is an alternative psychotherapeutic modality, stating that when we press certain points along a subject's meridians while he is thinking of a negative emotion, his being is brought back to the state of equilibrium, because his/her attention to negative emotions in the same old way is distracted, while new ones are chosen from the expanded unconscious possibilities and materialized in the form of a new association. You can see the similarity of this technique with acupuncture. EFT practitioners say that this technique can heal depression, anxiety, dependency or phobias. However, if the emotional wound is too deep and the therapy does not completely heal, there is chakra psychology.

OPENING THE BLOCKED CHAKRAS

Still one step deeper than psychoanalytic therapy, or even energy psychology techniques, is chakra psychology. Chakra psychology uses psychotherapy to remove blockage or imbalance of vital energy at individual chakras.

Some psychologists go too far in suggesting that all diseases have one ultimate reason; we cause them through confusion of our intentions. But we can't; in our ego we do not have the power of intention or downward causation. Instead, what happens is that our conditioned thoughts inappropriately amplify the movement of vital energy in and out of the chakras, adding to already existing disharmony of the chakras. Chakra psychology attempts to harmonize this disharmony. Below, we provide a chakra-by-chakra description of how chakra psychology works (just a glimpse mind you; for further details, see Page's book *Frontiers of Health*).

I (Valentina) use hatha yoga quantum style with my students and with my patients, using the asanas (hatha yoga postures) for helping the creative process. There is no better way if people truly aim to "open" their chakras.

If the disease involves the root chakra (elimination systems), then the problem is insecurity, not enough healthy grounding. Remember, in the current culture we try to ground ourselves through watching sex and violence on TV, for example, which is an unhealthy way of grounding. What is healthy grounding? Simple tasks like gardening and walking barefoot on grass can help us get grounded, but this also means working with vital energy at the vital level. To work on the vital energy imbalance through the mind, we can use imagination and visualization. For example, close your eyes and imagine that there are red roots from your root chakra that extend all the way to the center of the Earth.

For the second chakra, we can use our sexual relationships to balance vital energy imbalance. Have you been ignoring your feminine side, if you are male, or your masculine side, if you are female, which Carl Jung discovered and named your *anima* and *animus*, respectively? To integrate the male and the female within you (which balances sexuality), during sexual union, visualize yourself as both male and female. This visualization practice can also be done even without sex.

For the navel chakra, how do you deal with the mental amplification of anger and irritation that becomes chronic? Your mental hurriedness and impatience are the major factors here. So the psychological work here is to slow down the mind via meditation.

Hostility is a contraction of the energy at the heart so the objective of psychotherapy at this chakra is to expand the heart. As Swami Sivananda, a spiritual master in India who lived in the last century, used to advise, "Be good, do good," as in simple acts of giving to the needy with goodness in heart. This expands the heart. Also, loving yourself makes you available to love others, for the energy does not leave the heart chakra; this banishes hostility.

Often other people's vital energy hits us at the heart chakra, producing a contraction of consciousness, especially when we are naturally sympathetic (recall the mirror neurons). If that is the case, we must try to be objective and not identify with the others' troubles, and yet remain loving, for which we invoke nonlocality (empathy training).

Visualization is of great help in dealing with suppression of vital energy at the heart, which produces immune system malfunction. You may visualize putting a reflector around your body to reflect back all the received vital energy whenever you interact with another of negative energy (it helps to put on shiny clothes while doing this exercise). You can visualize energetic killer T cells fighting with intruders in your body and winning the battle. In some human potential workshops, leaders demonstrate the efficacy of visualization by letting you visualize your headache and making it smaller and smaller. Indeed, for some people, the headache *is* literally visualized away. Guided imagery is routinely used for the relief of chronic pain and for accelerating healing and easing discomfort from injuries. Visualization is useful for working with chakras, in general.

How does visualization work? Visualization feeds seeds of new meaning with potentiality for further expansion in the unconscious, processing and enabling your consciousness to choose from a larger pool of new possibilities. This mainly refers to situational creativity in, but it is often quite effective.

For the throat chakra imbalance of vital energy, to deal with frustration of expression, the psychological task again is to find avenues for situational creativity to enter the picture. If avenues in the public arena are not available (not everybody is born with required talent), then engage in private, smaller arenas of creativity. For example, be creative in gardening, cooking, relating, singing in the shower, dancing to rock 'n' roll music, writing in a diary, drawing on paper, trying to understand scientific ideas, etc.

In dealing with the blockage of vital energy in the third eye having to do with suppression, the question to ask is, "What is this block keeping me from doing?" The answer, of course, is that it is keeping you from the full expression of your meaning possibilities by denying the facility of focusing. For example, when we have headaches, we cannot focus. Mentally, you are taking yourself and your learned repertoire of expertise too seriously. Lighten up. There are many more possibilities to explore, so learn to play with them.

New paradigm science conferences often include humor and laughter as regular activities. At the European transpersonal psychology conference in Assisi, Italy, in 2000, we participated in laughing meditation for half an hour every day. I (Valentina) use laughing meditation exercises for loosening up participants routinely in our quantum activism workshops.

To work with blocked energy at the brow and crown chakra, one of the best psychotherapeutic tools is a meditation on peace.

Working with all three chakras in the brain is very important.

Remember that song in the film *My Fair Lady*: "The rain in Spain stays mainly in the plain?" Here's a helpful new lyric set to the same tune: Appreciate that "the pain of strain is mainly in the brain." This is because of the brain's direct correlation with the mind. So we must do vital energy practices to augment the meditation on peace and take up practices such as hatha yoga, pranayama, Tai chi, etc.

A common method for healing all of the chakras is to regularly visualize healthy vital energy at each chakra. Do the chakra meditation described earlier with a partner. That meditation, which also involves a lot of visualization, can be used to heal the chakras.

CARING FOR THE MENTAL: THE INFORMATION LEVEL

In the current materialist culture, when doctors speak of strategies for good health, we include good hygiene, good nutrition, exercise, and regular check-ups (with a conventional medicine expert of course). They are really speaking of caring only for the physical body. In contrast, positive health begins when we start caring also for our vital, mental, supramental, and even bliss body.

What does good hygiene for the vital or mental body mean? Just as physical hygiene tells us to avoid harmful physical environments, similarly, vital and mental hygiene must mean avoiding vital and mental pollution. And information and social media is mental pollution—a little of it unavoidable, but do too much, that will hurt you.

The following episode appeared in the comic strip *Dilbert*. Dilbert says to one of his coworkers, "My digital devices have reduced my attention span so much I can barely concentrate on work." In the next frame he continues, "I need a dopamine hit every four seconds or I look for something else to do." What is his colleague's response to all this? "Would you mind terribly if I play with my phone while you drone on and on?"

Yes, it's funny, but it's also sad. When I hear somebody say that the

Internet has given him a respite from boredom, I shudder. Yes, but at what cost?

CARING FOR THE MENTAL: THE MEANING LEVEL

Nutrition of the mental means feeding ourselves good literature, good music, poetry, art, what normally is called soul food, which is no less important than regular food. Entertainment that provokes laughter and joy is to be preferred to that which makes you feel "heavy." That is the general rule of mental nutrition.

How do we exercise the mental? For the mental body, the exercise is concentration—for example, mentally repeating a mantra such as *Om*. You can practice it during work, or you can sit and do concentration meditation as in Transcendental Meditation practice.

Occasional creative quantum leaps are important for the mental body, because only then does the mind get to process truly new meaning because of the new context involved. There is a story about the Impressionist artist Rene Magritte. He was walking down the street one day when a display cake in a confectioner's window side-tracked him. He went inside and asked for the cake. But when the shopkeeper brought out the cake in the display case, Magritte objected. "I want another one." "Why?" the shopkeeper asked. Magritte answered, "I don't want the display cake because people have been looking at it." Likewise, it is healthier for your mind to not always process only those thoughts that everyone is processing. Hence, the importance of creativity.

Finally, some very good news from the empirical front: Neuroscientists have found that long-term meditation does increase the happiness level. It is the job of neuroscientists to develop neuroscience signatures of happiness. In the 1970s, the researchers Richard Davidson and Daniel Goleman consolidated their earlier work to point out one measure of happiness. Brain structures usually exist on both sides of the brain, as both the left and right hemisphere have a prefrontal cortex. And here is the signature: activity in the prefrontal cortex in the left hemisphere (LPFC) is correlated with positive affect—happiness; and a shift of activity to the right (RPFC) signifies negative affect—unhappiness. Indeed, research shows that long-term meditators pass this happiness test hands-down.

MEDITATION

At the next level of sophistication, we look into the cause of the behavior that is causing the health problem. At that level, we are ready to deal with the cause of our behavior, the mind-brain doshas: excessive intellectualism and excessive attention deficit and hyperactivity.

How do we deal with excessive intellectualism? Well, intellectualism keeps us away from the body, away from experiencing the emotions. Emotions become something of a nuisance, something to be ashamed of, something to suppress at all costs. As James Joyce wrote in one of his short stories, "A Painful Case": "Mr. Duffy lives a little distance from his body." This is the way all intellectuals live their lives. The remedy is, of course, to indulge in the body. Exercise is good, massage is good, even simply hugging people is good.

I (Amit) myself was an intellectual many years ago. When I was doing intense spiritual work in the eighties, the brain/mind dosha of intellectualism, although not yet a health problem, became a problem because it blocked my spiritual opening. I remember going to a workshop and the workshop leader (the physician Richard Moss) prescribed "juicy physicality," for me to be administered as hugs from my fellow workshop attendees. It worked.

A complementary technique is meditation with the purpose of becoming aware of feelings so as not to suppress them with defense mechanisms or rationalization. Intellectuals are good in concentration or focused activity. So concentration meditation—for example, repeating a mantra mentally—comes naturally to intellectuals. To be aware of their dosha pattern, they must additionally practice relaxed witnessing, and watch everything to come in the inner awareness without judgment, including the watcher, just as a witness is supposed to do with courtroom evidence.

How does one work with excessive hyperactivity? The basic objective here is to slow down.

Do an experiment. Take a coffee break right now while you are reading this book. No hurry, the book is not going to run away. Make the coffee as part of a ritual, paying attention to every step. When the coffee is prepared, sit down with a cup of it. Slowly lift the cup to your mouth and take a sip. Watch the response: "Ah..." You feel relaxed, you feel happy.

It is easy to rationalize away: Happiness is a good cup of coffee. But a little experimentation will easily convince you that happiness is not inherent in the coffee, but instead came from the momentary expansion of your consciousness. Slowing down, first and foremost, is a way to expand our consciousness that produces happiness, bliss.

Now you can see what hyperactivity is depriving you from: bliss. And the more you indulge in hyperactivity, the more it robs you of bliss. First comes sleeplessness. Sleep is bliss, being in unbroken consciousness. Then come relationship problems: more separateness and less bliss. Finally, the disease: separateness has risen to a maximum. Slowing down single-handedly makes room for the dissolution of separateness.

In 1991, I (Amit) was invited to a yoga conference in India to give a talk on consciousness and quantum physics and I was, generally speaking, taking myself a bit too seriously. Then one of the teachers there asked me, "What do you do when you are by yourself?" And my psychological inflation came crashing down. I had to admit to myself that when I was by myself, I was fidgety and bored, always trying to find something to do. I realized that I needed to slow down.

How does one slow down? You can only take so many coffee breaks in a day. Also coffee, which contains caffeine, increases hyperactivity. The primary answer here is also meditation, but the approach to meditation is different.

Hyperactivity in children is common in this country and such children often suffer from attention deficit disorder. This is, of course, when hyperactivity is already pathological, but attention deficit is a common associate of hyperactivity even for adults. So hyperactive people must learn to focus their attention which is the objective of usual forms of meditation called concentration meditation, such as repeating mentally a mantra over and over as in Transcendental Meditation. It helps initially to learn to concentrate on other objects as well, such as on a candle flame, on the breath, and so forth.

Meditation in this concentrated form has now become famous as causing the "relaxation response," thanks to Herbert Benson's pioneering research; this is the topic of his book *The Relaxation Response*.

Do a little practice. Sit comfortably, close your eyes, breathe evenly, and repeat a common mantra such as the Sanskrit word "Om" in your mind. Of course your mind will find distractions, but as soon as you discover a distraction, bring your mind firmly back to the mantra. Do it for five minutes.

Now open your eyes. How many times did you move away from your mantra? Five times? Twenty-five times? It is hard, isn't it? It is a lot of work. So, be prepared. It takes some serious practice to quiet the mind enough to hold attention for a time.

QUANTUM YOGA FOR THE MIND

Still further in sophistication and subtlety are techniques that deal with the root of the mind-brain doshas and the misuse of the mental *gunas* themselves. Remember that the doshas are produced by the unbalanced application of the gunas, the mental qualities we are born with. If we can balance the qualities of sattva and rajas (and also tamas—inertia—since often we do not use tamas enough when sattva and rajas dominate our persona), then the mind-brain doshas will no longer haunt us.

In principle, it is easy. People of sattva have to engage more in problems of the ordinary world and ordinary living, which requires only rajasic skills and natural tamas. And people of rajas have to be more interested in fundamental creativity, in the context of thinking itself, in the archetypal domain of love, beauty, and justice. And both kinds of people, sattvic and rajasic, must practice with relaxation, balancing tamas in their life. They need to make do-be-do-be-do their lifestyle.

In practice, these balancing tricks constitute the heart of yoga. The objective of yoga is to integrate the separate self, the ego, and the universal unity of the quantum self. Why involve the quantum self in healing? Consciousness has only one way of manifesting its purposiveness in the world, and that one way is the creative freedom of choice, for choosing the new from among the quantum possibilities the unique actuality of manifest creative insight. But this creative freedom is the domain of the quantum self. We have free will to heal ourselves only to the extent we are able to precipitate the act of healing in our quantum self-consciousness. Hence, yoga is paramount.

Since sattva or fundamental creativity takes us beyond the mind, using the quality of sattva is already a yoga; it is called *jnana* (meaning wisdom) yoga. Rajas, on the other hand, is the tendency to use the discoveries of sattva to worldly purposes of empire building, employing situational creativity, and problem-solving skills. Rajas can be used for selfish personal aggrandizement, which just serves the ego. If, however, the acts of rajas are done with selflessness for the good of the world, then these acts become yoga also. It is called karma (in this context meaning action) yoga. In truth, karma yoga is better done in the service of love, and the yoga of cultivation of love is called *bhakti* (meaning love) yoga.

So the balancing act for the person of excessive sattva is to continue to practice jnana yoga with some karma yoga and bhakti yoga. And the balancing act for the person of rajas is to practice karma yoga in conjunction with jnana and bhakti yoga.

There is also another balancing that needs to be done: the balancing of the mind, the vital, and the physical. This is called raja yoga, which was codified by the great yogi Patanjali. Raja yoga incorporates hatha yoga—physical postures, and pranayama, breathing practices. Needless to mention, in the West the combination of hatha yoga and pranayama is what is called yoga. But the goal of raja yoga is to integrate the action of the physical body, the energy body, and the mental body so that the ego can integrate with the quantum self. So the beginning practices of hatha yoga and pranayama are complemented by the practices of meditation as well in the service of creative quantum leaps.

To repeat: If you have practiced any hatha yoga postures, your first impression may be that it is just stretching exercise. However, you are missing a point or two. First, hatha yoga postures have to be done slowly, so consciousness expands while doing the stretching. Second, in hatha yoga, one must pay attention to the internal goings on, especially to the flow of vital energy. The second objective of hatha yoga is practiced more directly in pranayama or breathing practices. Notice also that paying attention to the breath has the effect of slowing it down, and thus slowing down the activity of our internal organs.

THE SUPRAMENTAL BODY (INTUITIVE LEVEL)

Nourishment for the supramental level involves focusing on:

1. Engaging in the intuitions—intuitive thoughts and noble feelings.
2. Engaging situational creativity to follow up the intuitions via the creative process. This will be much facilitated by adapting the do-be-do-be-do lifestyle, an emphasis on doing interspersed with relaxation and let-go, a concept that we introduced before.
3. Engaging the flow experience.

In our workshops we both often lead participants in a flow meditation by following an idea that originally came from the Christian mystic Brother Lawrence (1614-1691), a simple-minded and good-hearted cook who engaged in what he called "practicing the presence of God to attain enlightenment."

In our version of this practice, you begin by sitting comfortably and doing a quick body awareness exercise to bring the vital energy down to the body from the active brow chakra. Next, you bring love energy to your heart. You can do this in a variety of ways. Think of a loved one (your primary relationship) or a revered one (for example, Jesus, Buddha, Mohammed, or Ramana Maharshi), or simply think of God's love. Once you feel the energy in your heart, diffuse your attention (like you do when you move from focused eyes to "soft" eyes). Let some of your attention go to peripheral activities that are going on around you—sounds, sights, even chores. Let there become a flow between your soft attention at the heart (being) and the stuff at the periphery (doing). Imagine yourself taking a shower with a shower cap on. The water wets you everywhere, but not your hair. Similarly, the worldly chores grab your attention away from feelings at all the chakras, but never from your heart. Once you get a hang of it, you can do what Brother Lawrence did, and live your life in flow.

REMEMBERING DHARMA

The discovering and fulfilling of our personal dharma will make us more authentic and, at the same time, better able to find the necessary resources to solve any problems. Each of us has an extraordinary unique divine gift which confers us our unicity and the reason for which we incarnated. Too many of us, unfortunately, sacrifice this divine gift on the altar of conformism and mimetism. The way we react to events and the way we aspire towards certain ideals is and will always remain unique.

As Yogi Berra once said, "If you don't know where you are going, you might wind up someplace else." In reality, not knowing our essential destination means to ignore our own purposeful mission in the universe and to serve other people's purpose or woes—other people's me-centered pursuits—and this acute state of ignorance will lead us toward another direction than the one toward which our soul aspires (even when our mind doesn't realize it yet). When we do that, everything is in the direction of our dharma—and everything that is wonderful and divine inside of us will blossom. When we listen to this call of our Heart, we also discover the immense resources through which we can alchemize and transform all our problems and obstacles. Transformation will start from inside, and its echoes will be heard more or less on the outside as well.

Our dharma is a confluence between our deepest heart yearnings and the most important requirements of the external reality; when both aspects are in harmony, we don't have the sensation of making effort in our archetypal explorations.

Confucius said: "The moment you found your life mission and you can have the profession that your heart truly wants, you will never work again, not even for a single day." Work then becomes play—*lila*, a celebration, such a beautiful and fascinating activity that we will not feel it as an effort.

NOURISHING THE BLISS BODY

Developing sensitivity to intuitions and following up your intuitions through fundamental creativity is the way to keep your bliss body (the quantum self and the wholeness beyond) nourished.

For the bliss body, the lazy person's exercise is sleep. But when we wake from sleep, although sometimes we do feel happy, we always remain the same even though during sleep we enjoyed being without the subject-object split. This is because the likelihood is that only our habitual patterns of possibilities of our personal unconscious are available for consciousness to process during ordinary sleep.

I (Valentina) always emphasize mental hygiene to my clients and students of quantum yoga. Any negativity that you cling to will surface in your dreams and make your sleep restless. My father's specializations in medicine were very much related to prevention, including preventive medicine, hygiene of the physical environment, including radiation hygiene. In that line of thought, he developed his intuition while he was practicing general medicine, and towards the last years of his life, he also realized the importance of mental and emotional hygiene, thanks to my prompting. Likewise, I have learned from his example that being a doctor is truly a wonderful profession and a meaningful way of living.

This changes when we learn to sleep with creativity in mind. Then, states can be reached that are sleeplike, but when we wake up, we burst with inner creativity, and we may even transform. This "creative sleep" is the best exercise for the bliss body.

chapter fourteen

PREVENTIVE MEDICINE LESSON 5: QUANTUM YOGA FOR QUANTUM HEALING

Mind-body disease consists of chronic ailments in which the imposition of wrong mental meaning sets up disharmony in our vital and physical bodies. Specifically, the wrong mental meaning forces people to forget the higher physiology already attained by our ancestors and available to all for the heart and navel chakra organs.

You cannot correct a problem by staying at the same level that created the problem. So, mind-body healing involves changes in the meaning-context that the mind sets up for the malfunctioning of our vital and physical bodies.

The context of right mental thinking comes from the supramental domain of consciousness in the form of the archetype of wholeness; to change the context to a new right one, we mental beings will have to leap to the supramental. This leap is a discontinuous quantum leap of fundamental creativity, which is why this type of healing is called quantum healing.

The phrase "quantum healing" was creatively intuited by the physician Deepak Chopra, but the explanation he gave was tentative. In *The Quantum Doctor*, quantum healing was shown to be the culmination of the creative process. In this book, new knowledge of the self-identities at the heart and navel chakras enables us to construct a much more detailed map of what is involved.

FUNDAMENTAL CREATIVITY IN HEALING

What we call the wisdom of the body, illustrated spectacularly by the placebo effect, is an example of self-healing but it is ritualized in us: All you need to do is keep your healing intension active. If you lose it, faith in a doctor's word as in placebo healing rekindles your healing intension and should give you a glimpse of your own healing capacity. To truly manifest the entire scope of this capacity, the entire program of creativity, it is essential to go through all the stages of the creative process which ends in no less than a quantum insight about the change of context one has to make in one's living style. This insight itself is so powerful that often a quick healing of the affected organ takes place. However, to make the healing long-lasting, one also has to live up to the insight gained and institute the new lifestyle; make no mistake about it.

Since the new insight sought is about an archetype, it can also be approached from the vital plane, adding more punch to the process. For engaging vital creativity, the patient needs to concentrate on the chakra involved in the disease where the energy is blocked.

Suppose that instead of a belief that they are getting some sort of healing from somebody else as in placebo effect, patients operate under the conviction (a "burning" one because of the urgency of the situation) that they already have in potentiality the new software—mental and vital—for healing the physiology which they only need to discover and then implement in their lifestyle.

Since there is an emergency now, maintaining healing intension posits no problem for most people. Now begins the creative process: do-be-do-be-do and all that.

The first step of creative healing is preparation. Patients would be encouraged to research their disease (with a lot of help from their physicians, of course, who will act more as collaborators with empathy) and meditate on it. Such meditation will readily show the patients the role of brain-mind doshas as to how they deal with emotional stress, and how their habits of mentalization of feelings and suppression or expression of emotions as the case may be, contribute to the disease. One of the root causes of emotional stress accumulation will also become clear: do-do-do speed—hurrying and rushing—augmenting the pursuit of desires with accomplishment-orientation, anxieties and day dreaming. So the first purpose of the preparation stage is to slow down the mental and vital conscious processing and to create an open, receptive attitude that is an essential first step toward any creativity.

At the next stage, the patients and their doctors would try various techniques of mind-body medicine—yoga, pranayama, chi gong, etc. (These may be new to the patient in which case the healer may have to play the role of teacher as well.) This is also the stage of creativity in which we use unlearned stimuli and divergent thinking to generate previously uncollapsed possibility waves of the vital, mental, and the supramental that expand in the unconscious; but we don't show preference among the conscious possibilities we generate. Since only choice of downward causation can create an event of conscious awareness, what is involved is unconscious processing—processing without awareness. In other words, this stage is the combination of alternate preparation and incubation—do-be-do-be-do.

There are well-known cases of art therapy, in which patients attempt to heal themselves by submerging into beautiful, spiritual art, preferably created by their own healing imagination. Art therapy does not work for everybody. But how does art therapy work at all, even for some people? When art is inspired by the imagination of healing emotions, very soon conscious processing gives way to unconscious processing as well, and it is the do-be-do-be-do that inspires further art and opens up new vista of healing possibilities.

Similarly, certain yoga postures accompanying visualization suitably designed with evocative healing archetypal images will accomplish the same thing—produce new possibilities of vital feelings and mental thinking for consciousness to choose from.

Do-be-do-be-do style movement—alternating movement such as dancing or Tai chi with the relaxation of healing meditation—works too.

Sooner or later, a seemingly inconsequential trigger precipitates the quantum leap of insight. Spontaneously, a new supramental context and the vital-mental gestalt that represents it appear manifest in conscious awareness. The insight leads to the corrective contextual shift of how the mind handles emotions. The initial manifestation of the insight begins at once: Freed from the shackles of mentalization, as the new liturgical fields are experienced, the old software programs and the organ physiology itself become functional once again at a healthy level, sometimes quite dramatically.

There are some reported successes in treating cancer patients via the use of creative visualization, for which the above scenario applies. Here is a particularly poignant description of one person's quantum healing through visualization; this story is taken from *The Healing Path* by the author Marc Barasch. A patient writes:

> When I was in Mexico, I had started having pain in my chest. I went across the border and got an MRI scan, which showed a mass on my thymus connecting to the aorta. I decided just to wait, but a scan six months later showed it was still there.
>
> I decided to spend a week at Carl Simonton's healing center in California, and I imaged "sharks eating cancer cells" as they recommended. But toward the end of the week, I had this extremely vivid, spontaneous vision that wasn't on the program. I saw a mass on my thymus as a piece of ice that just started to melt in these big, amazing drops. I've never in my life had this kind of clear image just come up by itself. And I knew instantly the drops are just teardrops. My whole life, through all the losses, I'd never been able to cry. Now there

was this melting away of the oppression I'd been feeling; the deaths and the abuse in my childhood, the unresolved relationship with my ex-husband. The emotion was suddenly available, and it felt so powerful.

Four months later, I had another MRI, and the mass was gone—there was no sign of it. I had no new treatment. Whatever this mass had been, they said the only way they could tell it had ever been there was from the previous two tests. —Marc Barasch, *The Healing Path*, pp. 273-274

Such experiences vary. The example above was a vision. In his book *The Black Butterfly*, the physician Richard Moss talks of a cancer patient who attended one of his workshops. During the workshop, she was defiant and was not responding to the various attempts of Moss to energize her. But at some point Moss broke through her shell and she responded by participating in a spontaneous dance that led to a dramatic *ah-ha* experience. The following morning the patient woke up feeling so much better that Moss sent her for a checkup. Her cancer was gone.

The patient in Moss's anecdote experienced the more usual ah-ha of creative insight, but a quantum leap in the vital domain initiated the process. Patients also report experiencing the choice itself, when the purity of the healing intention is crystallized. As an example, here is the physician Deepak Chopra's account, from his book *Quantum Healing*, of the healing of a cancer patient through sudden insight:

... a quiet woman in her fifties came to me about ten years ago complaining of severe abdominal pains and jaundice. Believing that she was suffering from gallstones, I had her admitted for immediate surgery, but when she was opened up, it was found that she had a large malignant tumor that had spread to her liver, with scattered pockets of cancer throughout her abdominal cavity.

Judging the case inoperable, her surgeons closed the incision without taking further action. Because the woman's daughter pleaded with me not to tell her mother the truth, I informed my patient that the gallstones had been successfully removed. I rationalized that her family would break the news to her in time...

Eight months later I was astonished to see the same woman back in my office. She had returned for a routine physical exam, which revealed no jaundice, no pain, and no detectable sign of cancer. Only after another year passed did she confess anything unusual to me. She said, "Doctor, I was so sure I had cancer two years ago that when it turned out to be just gallstones, I told myself I would never be sick another day in my life." Her cancer never returned.

This woman used no technique; she got well, it appears, through her deep-seated resolve, and that was good enough.... I must call it a quantum event, because of the fundamental transformation that went deeper than organs, tissues, cells, or even DNA, directly to the source of body's existence in time and space. —Deepak Chopra, *Quantum Healing*, pp. 102-103

So it is easy to conclude that spontaneous healing of cancer is due to the sudden onset of such a dynamic surge in immune system activity that the cancerous growth is gotten rid of within days, even hours. The use of the creative process makes this kind of healing by quantum leaping available for every patient.

To repeat, the immune system malfunction is due to faulty vital and mental processing—excessive mentalization, intellectualism, suppression of love energy at the heart chakra, taking its toll. A quantum leap to the supramental is accompanied by a shift of mental meaning and the unblocking of love energy at the heart chakra. This then can have the desired dynamic effect on the immune system in the form of reactivating its software program of getting rid of cancerous cells with such vigor as to effect very rapid healing.

The final stage of the creative process—manifestation—is also important to discuss in this creative quantum healing. Manifestation is not complete with only the reactivation of vital programs that are needed for the normal functioning of the organ(s) involved. Remember the vital-physical and mind-brain doshas are still there. After the remission has taken place, the patient has to bring to manifestation using the new insight some of the life style changes that are commensurate with the shift of context of mental processing and the processing of feelings if the remission is to be stable and permanent. For example, a lifestyle that produces excessive intellectualism and defensive reactions must give way to a more balanced one that allows love to manifest regularly.

Why do most placebo healing cases appear to be only temporary healing? The faith that "I am getting medicine from my doctor whom I trust" leads a reactivation of the patient's healing intention and consciousness responds with a reshuffling of known meaning contexts of the mind that temporarily allows the mind and the vital-physical organs to make the necessary changes. In other words, they are examples of healing due to situational creativity. Such situational adjustments are not adequate for long because the situation keeps on changing.

Can the idea of quantum healing via the creative process be invoked by anyone? A physician in Bangalore, India, named Dr. B. Monappa Hegde, M.D., took it upon himself to verify it and heal his retinal edema. This is documented. Dr. Hegde and Amit wrote a joint paper on the subject.

Q & A

Authors: But if consciousness chooses, and consciousness is us, why don't we always choose "health?" Why do we suffer from illness or disease at all?

Quantum Physicist: Ah, the quintessential subtlety of choice. In the seventies, Fred Alan Wolf created the New Age slogan, "We create our own reality." He meant well but was much misunderstood. People first tried to manifest porches you know, following Wolf's dictum. They did not succeed, so they tried to manifest parking spaces for their cars for a while and be content with that.

But, kidding aside, in our ordinary ego, we are ignorant and conditioned to suffer due to the ignorance of our healing power. Choice always happens from the possibilities that are available. When we are in our ego, only the conditioned possibilities are available with large probability, so the creative choice to wellness is easily missed.

Authors: So, once we are ill, a quantum leap is necessary if we want to heal ourselves using self-healing only.

Quantum physicist: This is so. This is what Mary Baker Eddy missed, and so Christian Science to this day invites disaster for many of its practitioners by forbidding medical help entirely. Not everyone is ready for quantum leaps acting solo to discover a new contextual meaning of the wholeness archetype. For them, medicinal systems, limited as they are, are better prescriptions.

And moreover, creative healing would be well-nigh a miracle if the disease is at the physical level only. It is one thing if Christian Science confined itself to mind-body healing. But the blanket imposition of such high-level demands of creativity to all diseased parishioners even suffering from a bacterial infection is foolhardy.

QUANTUM YOGA

We have developed a deeply transformational program called Quantum Yoga. A big part of it refers to Health maintenance and Healing. The overall experiential goal of quantum yoga is the ability to live and act from expanded inclusive states of consciousness.

The anecdotes cited above each suggest a quantum yoga healing exercise for removing heart chakra energy block.

1. Do-be-do-be-do with visualization.
    Lie down comfortably (*shavasana*—corpse posture) and visualize that your heart and chest area is frozen as if there are some blocks of ice surrounding the heart chakra. Feel the heaviness and the cold of the ice. After a while, imagine that the ice is

melting and becoming teardrops, teardrops of relief of the grief for all the suppressed love in your life.

2. Do-be-do-be-do: alternative dancing and resting
   This is done in four steps:
   1. Shake all parts of your body thoroughly for a few minutes.
   2. Let somebody shout STOP. You stop at once and freeze in that position in awareness meditation.
   3. Again, somebody shouts DANCE. Begin dancing slowly at first but picking up speed and vigor with time putting you whole mind to it paying attention to movements of energy in the upper body.
   4. Then somebody says MEDITATE. Sit down in *bajarasana* (kneeling down sitting on your feet). Meditate on well-being.

The final episode above suggests the importance of the purity of your healing intention. Purity of intention is crucial for quantum leaps of fundamental creativity, all creativity. Our creativity is illusive because our intentions are so conflicted, so confused. However, the good news is that you can do a practice to develop your power of intention. It consists of several stages:

1. You start making the intention of healing from your ego; this is where you are. However, use healing art or music to inspire you. That is, you intend for healing for yourself, healing for your particular disease, but from an expanded consciousness.
2. At the second stage, let your egoic intention for healing yourself be generalized to the intention of healing all. After all, if everyone is healed, you are included too.
3. At the third stage, let your intention become more like a prayer:

let the healing take place if it is in accordance with the purposive movement of consciousness.
4. At stage four, let the prayer sink into silence and become a meditation.

chapter fifteen

PREVENTIVE MEDICINE LESSON 6:
GOING DEEP IN YOUR PRACTICE FOR QUANTUM HEALING

One reason people get ill is because they don't dare to live. Then an illness sneaks in and the big problem is not that one gets ill. The big problem is that when illness comes, people become paralyzed by it. The biggest fear people have when the illness comes is that they are hopeless; they cannot do anything to heal.

Imagine you're suffering a disease and you don't know how to heal yourself and, additionally, you don't have the right perspective. Well, it is like this because basically you live this narrow perspective of life in a homeostasis—the base-level human condition; you don't need to go further you assume. So, you don't give enough, you don't expand enough, you don't think you have any resources like the infinite potentialities that quantum physics promises, and that is why when an illness comes it's very difficult for you to face it.

In a generous soul, which is also, by the way, a very optimistic soul, you look for and find new possibilities. Any illness can be healed. As you've got there, you will get out of there, no problem if you know how to heal. You always have a horizon, a perspective ahead. Even dying is a possibility which you can take into consideration very generously. "All right, this will be my last adventure. Shall I exit after that last scene on the stage? Let's see how that works." There are people who have tried this and what happened is that in the last moment the quantum leap of healing takes place as if the quantum self said, "Actually, enough suffering. It is enough, it was just another intensive experience of your very intense life. Get back to work now because you and I have a lot more to do."

There is a parable which says: "In hell there are tables filled with food but very huge spoons. And people starve because they can't use these big spoons. In heaven, the tables are set the same way with a lot of food and large spoons, but people feed each other with the spoons."

If a person comes to me (Valentina) for quantum healing with the idea: "What if it doesn't work?" I wouldn't start healing with such a person. That's because it's meaningless—you can do nothing to help. Even if I were to equivocate—"I can try to heal you, but let's see if it works; if it doesn't, I have something else for you"—it would compromise the situation. For instance, in case of the breast cancer, doctors are always telling women, "Check your breasts for lumps; check yourself every month." Of course, if you check for lumps all the time, you will probably end up finding one.

So before transforming this attitude, we cannot talk about a real quantum healing. It's an entire process: Fixing this one thing will actually fix most of the problems, you don't need anything more. You cannot imagine for example how many problems, especially related to the area of the chest are solved just by teaching people to be generous. It's immediate. It works, rapidly. To be generous, to give, to give, to give—no problem, give everything and then there is no problem left.

A process of healing starts with becoming aware of what we are and what we do, the resonances we experience with the archetypes, and so on. It is a question of authenticity, you see: Most of our health problems are generated by a difference of perception between what we really are and what we think we are, what reality is and how we cognize it. These two things conflict each other and create illness. When we've solved that one, there remains very little—only bones to fix and things like that.

How do we deepen the connection with the quantum self? Make the quantum self into your personal God. Then connect to it by praying, by even orienting our love toward that God within. This way of relationship with God is something very dynamic; it is the most dynamic relationship we'll ever have, because it can transform us the most. A person having a relationship with a personal God is a person who accepts the idea of healing and transformation. When God enters our life this way, life becomes a continuous journey of creativity and transformation. Quantum healing can take place regularly. When creativity stops, when transformation stops, death appears.

Therefore, a person who has a relationship with a personal God is a person who is ready for life. A person who is afraid of life is a person who is afraid of God, a person who doesn't have a personal relationship with God, a person who's running away from God and reality. We must have a personal relationship with God. To relate with your own deep self is not religion—this is not dogma or unnecessary belief.

When we doctors and healers attempt to heal somebody, that is the first thing we have to heal in our patients: Their relationship with God must be made personal. Of course, for avowed atheists, it is better to use the concept of Oneness than use the word God.

What happens when we have a personal relationship with God is that with ongoing states of ecstatic communion with God in the form of quantum self, we are inspired to engage in soul-making. This is when we engage fundamental creativity, we approach the archetypal realm, and quantum healing comes from that archetypal supramental level of our being. In the beginning, these communions are short and weak, but they grow constantly, and then, because of our communion with God becoming stronger, there occur some permanent effects of this: a life of ongoing creativity and transformation.

For example, because we have access to infinite potentiality, we no longer play the zero-sum game in which your gain must come from my loss and vice versa. Instead of competing, now we become infinitely generous. The less we are in contact with God, the more we become stingy. We feel poor, we feel alone, like little helpless creatures in an immense universe which is chaotic to boot. In addition, if we want to collect any last drop of pleasure, any last drop of happiness that we access, then the more we try, the more that happiness slips away through our fingers—because, of course, that is the lesson. Consciousness created the whole science of manifestation this way in order to make it possible for everyone, even those who need to be hit by the two-by-four of sickness into the exploration of its quantum potentialities.

Also, by feeling in an ongoing manner, more and more often, the presence of the divine spirit within our being, we will be more and more unlimited in the way we love and engage wholeness, the archetype of health.

Unconditionality. We will be able to love without conditions, without putting any conditions to ourselves: "I will love this person, if this happens." "I will love if I have that…." "I will love, if it is in this way." We will just simply love, and that love, as we have shown before, will lead to the fact that we discover the source of the happiness—expansion of consciousness—not that condition with which we love, which we mistake with the source of happiness. And this is the answer to how we can love without any limits. Love without any limits is already the perfect background for healing; actually, it rebalances our being automatically.

All in all, we can say that this is the key: To bring a personal God into our life is essential for complete quantum healing. Actually, this is the real source of suffering of the human being: not being aware of this Presence, the presence of a personal God, looking over us. We create the illusion of being separated, being independent and separate; this is our big melodrama. Everything else is just a projection outside of our inner melodrama. We behave like a child who is screaming but doesn't accept the mother's embrace because he is actually screaming for the mother's affection. But he doesn't know what to do and he is kicking around; he will be screaming until, finally exhausted from crying, he relaxes and falls into the arms of his mother.

So this is actually what happens when sometimes people are severely ill. That's why you will find among the terminal-phase patients a few people who are miraculously healed, but actually the first thing they may describe is the fact that they saw light, that they felt this extraordinary peaceful, harmonizing, divine energy, and then, suddenly the illness was gone, and their life begins to transform.

When we speak about self-healing using quantum creativity, we have to develop, in the first phase, and implement an objective, detached, and lucid way to see the disease. We have to be firm yet optimistic and to see the possibility that the disease may be a consequence of the mistakes we once made and acknowledge that maybe, in some sense, we created our disease. That's the first step.

Seeing the disease as the effect of your wrong lifestyle will open you to new possibilities for exploration and use a lot of methods to create different alternative resonances in your being—methods such as of medicinal herbs, acupuncture, chakra healing, music and art therapy, hypnotherapy, meditation and similar techniques, and if they do not fully work, engage quantum creativity, do-be-do-be-do, and the creative process. That's the second step.

And the second step—the creative process of fundamental creativity—crucially requires developing a character trait that is a big lack these days. It's called perseverance. In the second step we have to visualize constantly, firmly, repeatedly that we are healthy, that we are having very good resonances with the archetypes we are exploring and thus expansions of consciousness—we have to visualize ourselves in a very harmonious state. That creative, firm visualization has to be practiced even if we are feeling down, even if the quantum leap is not coming in a hurry, even if we feel completely smashed by our failure to make progress. Visualization and active imagination are miraculous when followed by relaxation, by unconscious processing of the possibilities that visualization brings us. But we have to practice this do-be-do-be-do with resilience, constantly reminding us that failures are the pillars of success.

A responsible person will pay the price because she realizes what she gets. The miraculous thing is that while you get healed by something, in reality you get healed by lots of other things which you didn't even realize were connected with the illness. So, in reality, when the spiritual healing process ends—when you can say, "Now I'm healed"—in reality, you are in a much higher consciousness than you were before starting the process of healing because you're healing lots of things which were connected with the visible illness and which you hadn't spotted. So, therefore the process of healing is not like people usually believe: "Oh, come on, I just have to heal this little flu and it should take no more than a week."

A part of your mind will say: "Oh, I don't even like this theory. Perseverance, my elbow. I want to heal faster; I want it now!" That part of your mind is sorry that it bought into the "I create my own reality" nonsense. It wants that blue pill—just to swallow it, not to do all those complicated things.

Without perseverance, without resilience, quantum healing is not going to happen. No matter what kind of amazing methods we have, perseverance is the key here. You might ask yourself: "How can we increase the perseverance?" Well, first of all, you must develop the attitude of self-forgiveness. Forgive yourself for your failures. Second, don't take yourself so seriously. So, you bought into a whole bill of goods about the strength of your intentions, how they always manifest. They don't, you know, not when they require creativity. So develop humility.

In the final reckoning, the answer to how to be perseverant is amazingly simple: by persevering. This is how you increase the perseverance. When you persevere with surrender, consciousness responds with inspiration and resolve. To resonate, the practice is alternate intention and surrender.

DEEP MEDITATION

Why do we need steps and stages for the creative process to work? The probability of discovering a new idea or a new healed state of well-being is virtually zero. This is why spiritual wisdom is important: It is only God's Grace that takes you there. Why all the shenanigans then? To prove our sincerity, to demonstrate that we have really reached an impasse such as a conflict between two opposites that we cannot resolve. That is when we reach out to heaven, when we can say, "I am ready to go beyond the limits of human effort." Patanjali calls this process *Ishwara Pranidhana*.

Is there a way to bypass all these stages and go directly for God's Grace, Ishwara Pranidhana? Yes, there is, this is the royal road; actually, it's not a shortcut, but it is a very powerful way not only to precipitate a quantum leap of healing but also for solving even all the hidden health problems, the problems which haven't manifested as symptoms yet. Deep meditation, practiced systematically, not only keeps negative resonances at bay for us and makes us immune to all kind of strange influences, but also produces a conscious state of prolonged expansion of consciousness.

Deep meditation is the secret of healing. How do we usually practice awareness? We stay in awareness; we think about getting the positive resonance, it doesn't come. After a bit of this, we lose ourselves, we relax. After a time though, we think about how negative our resonances were before. Then again, we concentrate on awareness, on getting positive, get expanded, and again we think, "Hmm, yeah, I'm amazed how bad I was before, very bad, so bad I don't believe it." Again, we go back to the practice of awareness. With a lot of attention, we meditate on the positive resonances and then again comes that thought: "I can now see the difference, so let me focus on awareness, it works," and then after half an hour of this, we think, "Wow, I meditated half an hour. Lord, I did it; I sure have nailed awareness meditation."

This is not deep meditation. Deep meditation is when we reach a positive resonance and we just continue—we do not think, we do not evaluate, we just stay there. How long do we stay there? Maybe half an hour is enough, maybe five minutes; we do have worldly chores and duties of service. But the difference is really noticeable. When you come out of deep meditation, you don't go back to contraction either. Somehow, the negative resonances are more abated.

So, it does require training. It is not that easy to concentrate on getting a positive resonance and staying there for some time. It implies that you should train your mind if it doesn't work very easily, it implies a little bit of effort to train with this focusing and so on. We always prescribe a quantum leap or two of situational creativity to give us faith in the process.

Deep meditation is a royal path which indeed has miraculous healing powers, but it doesn't work that easily. I am talking about yogic meditation, the kind of meditation that the real pros do—meditation with loving kindness in the heart directly connecting to their personal God. We are not talking about just sitting and not moving the body or fidgeting or sitting with the eyes closed for an amount of time watching the thoughts go by like clouds in the sky without attachment until being distracted and going back to awareness—those are the usual practices. I've seen people sitting there for three hours, and nothing much to show for it except pain in the knees.

Experiments have been done in hospitals in India with patients trying deep meditation and many succeeded in healing diabetes and other diseases too. And the ones succeeding were the ones who really managed to get into deep meditation, a state of expanded consciousness, for a considerable period. This implies a lot of discipline and training on those patients' part; don't think it was easy.

The former *Saturday Review* editor Norman Cousins has written about his self-healing from the condition ankylosing spondylitis, a degenerative disease that causes the connective tissue in the spine to wither away. Experts estimated that his chance of recovery was one in five hundred. Cousins stopped standard medication and substituted it with mega doses of vitamin C, in full consultation with his physician. Most importantly though, he watched funny movies (mostly old W. C. Fields and the Marx brothers) and read his favorite comic books for an entire weekend. After this marathon weekend, Cousins is said to have completely recovered from his condition and resumed his very productive life.

Skeptics, of course, remain. There is a rumor that Cousins secretly used homeopathic medicine but was reluctant to admit it publicly. Could he have achieved and stayed in deep meditation with continual states of positive resonance the whole weekend? I think he not only could have, but very likely that is what he did. After all, no meditation needs to have a formal format.

"Pray as if everything depends on God and then act as if everything depends on you." —*St. Augustine* chapter sixteen

QUANTUM GERONTOLOGY: LIVE QUANTUM, LIVE HEALTHY, LIVE LONGER, DIE HAPPY

If you have ever read a book on old proverbs, maybe you remember this one: "The country who doesn't have old people should buy some." Or this one: "Old people are the wisest people; they have friendship with wisdom." But guess what? The opposite is true in our culture: Alzheimer's disease and other chronic conditions have become good friends with old people, replacing wisdom.

It was not so long ago that the first case of Alzheimer's was detected and now it is reaching epidemic proportions. These days, roughly 1 percent of Americans suffer from Alzheimer's disease, but the data is alarming because for the elderly aged over sixty-five, the rate of Alzheimer's deaths increased by an astounding 146 percent from 2000 to 2018. This should be a severe warning to humanity: Because people tend not to process meaning anymore, the repertoire of memory is not needed much either. Today's people are individualistic and defensive of their territory in their emotional relationships; this produces immune system inflammation that, in turn, contributes to the plaque on memory neurons consisting of amyloid beta protein deposits. This increasingly puts the memories out of the reach of conscious recall and eventually leads to the dementia that we call Alzheimer's disease. In this way, instead of growing older and wiser, people often grow older and demented.

What a way to end life. It causes a huge burden on society. So why is it happening? Because of the lack of a good science of health and a system of health education that teaches people how to live.

The million-dollar question is this: What will make people grow older and wiser? Lacking that, what is it that will guarantee the elderly quality of life and death with dignity? Obviously, unless there is a continuity of the quality of life as we age, what is longevity for?

In fact, the two outcomes—quality of life and longevity—are related. There is now conclusive evidence that living a purposive life leads to increased longevity. In our youth, we follow at least some purpose; life then is mainly spent in the service of the lower needs but engaging in professions allows people to entertain a modicum of archetypal explorations in their lives—abundance (businesspeople), power (politicians, leaders in general), truth (scientists, writers, poets, artists, some media persons), justice (some in the law profession), wholeness (healers, educators), etc. Unfortunately, the purpose of life then gets almost entirely tied up with one's professional life, so when people retire, their purpose and archetypes disappear from their life.

Quality of life, purpose, meaning—these are not in the purview of materialist science. Fortunately, even allopathic healers are not strict adherents of scientific materialism; they resort to the idea of evidence-based medicine to try out if meaning, purpose, love, spirituality, these nonmechanical things help the quality of life in elderly people under the guise of holistic medicine. These studies are generally all positive, so much so that some effort is being made—positive psychology is an example—to include, implicitly of course, the nonphysical in elderly care on a large scale. This is good news.

In affluent countries, in some professions, retirement is no longer compulsory. This is also good news for the elderly. But overall the materialist approach alone is grossly inadequate for healthcare of the elderly. Let's look at it at some detail.

The materialist approach to gerontology consists of sorting out the different contributions of three discernible factors:

1. the entropy problem: some amount of disorder enters people's lives due to their lifestyles;
2. illness, chronic or caused by accidents, bacteria and virus, especially the former; and
3. deterioration through normal aging.

The materialist treatment is of course allopathy—drugs mainly to cure disease, plus possibly a holistic approach to correct some of the lifestyle disorder causing emotional stress such as loneliness.

According to the American Holistic Health Association, "Holistic health is an approach to life that emphasizes the connection of the mind, body and spirit, with the goal of having everything functioning at its very best so you achieve maximum well-being. A key component to a holistic approach is taking responsibility for your well-being and making everyday choices that put you in charge of your health."

That sounds good, but the catch is that without an understanding of the nonmaterial nature of the mind and the spirit, and without accounting for vital feelings, the holistic medicine being developed is inadequate as well.

QUANTUM GERONTOLOGY

What can we do to help care for the elderly now that we have theory to guide us—quantum science in addition to evidence-based science? Quantum science's answer is: plenty. In effect, we are reformulating gerontology—elder care—into a quantum gerontology.

An article published in the *Journal of Gerontology* by Alexandra M. Freund, et al. claims that motivation is the key to healthy aging. Indeed, the difficulty with a lifestyle change from an unhealthy and sedentary one to a healthy and active one is motivation. It is easy to talk about simple maintenance exercises, which we have already mentioned in an earlier chapter. Many of these practices, such as yoga and meditation, have been around in some form or another for a long time. However, motivation is what keeps people from using the available knowledge. And, yes, let credit be given: Some of the recent awareness about this knowledge has been guided under the holism paradigm.

There is already an awareness as well in the humanistic-transpersonal-depth psychology models that human development is shaped by two psychological drives:

1. Hylotropy—a term used by psychiatrist Stan Grof to signify the drive toward ego-individuality and separateness; and
2. Holotropy—a drive toward wholeness, toward the quantum self, not for spiritual salvation or self-realization but for integration of all conflicts into a realization of the archetype of wholeness.

A study of human development shows that for most people, the call of hylotropy dominates. However, according to the quantum science of consciousness, there are two periods of exception that the Tibetans of ancient times called the *bardo*—a passageway for new exploration. One of these occurs at puberty and lasts through the teen years. The second one occurs at midlife, between ages forty and sixty, and is called the midlife transition. Because of the awakening of the drive toward holotropy, those people who do so awaken have extra motivation to make lifestyle changes. Quantum gerontology works best with this explicit awakening. The tasks of quantum gerontology are threefold:

1. To help people to grow old and wise, starting with the midlife transition through a protracted program that involves the embodiment of the archetypes via quantum science of manifestation and creativity at both mental and vital level—in other words, by engaging people in what we call the quantum yoga of soul-making. Some people, at midlife, contract chronic diseases

anyway because of past lifestyle abuses. This often generates added motivation for a healthy lifestyle during the aftermath of allopathic recovery.

2. To help people who recognize the call of holotropy but choose not to go through a midlife transition and instead revert back to the same-old with a reframing of their past and emphasize the positive. These people usually have chronic diseases later, especially after the age of sixty, and need therapeutic and medical care of some sort for the rest of their lives.

3. To help people who do not fall in either of the two categories above—that is, people who do not wake up to holotropy at midlife and let themselves deteriorate to what we call an "elderly problem" that needs caregiving in a nursing home or similar environment. The challenge is: Can we improve on the existing very poor treatment of this batch of elderly, which is by far the most common under the worldview-polarized materialist value-confused culture in which they live?

It is to the last category of people that holistic principles are being applied right now with some success and is a major opportunity for quantum entrepreneurship as well.

In the first category, people who are ready for soul-making are the primary interest of the quantum approach to life and living. In this chapter, we will concentrate on the first and second group of people, those who recognize the call of holotropy. We will discuss the aging issue and questions of longevity and outline a quantum integrative health strategy for these people.

In what way are the health practices different for older people than those discussed earlier as preventive medicine? Biological evolution gives us a set of universal physiological functions that we are born with, and that includes the mechanisms that dictate longevity and aging. The belief that dominates the biological community is that human physiology is permanent, and we cannot change the physiological functions of organs. Therefore, the effect of aging—for example, cell death—on the organs is bound to cause deterioration of organ functions.

Opposition to this idea has come from the quite ancient spiritual tradition of Tantra, which was first developed in India and then in Tibet. In Tantra, we find the mystical idea of kundalini—coiled-up energy at the lower chakras of root and sex—and its mysterious awakening—a rising up of the energy opening all the chakras higher up. Few people, however, reported having this awakening experience. Fewer yet have shown tangible signs of such "opening."

I (Amit) became curious about this phenomenon because I had an experience of opening while I was doing what seemed like a four-step exercise involving shaking the body, meditation, slow dancing, and another meditation session. In retrospect, after I developed a theory of mental creativity, I saw what I did as a do-be-do-be-do exercise in vital energy, and I began considering the idea that perhaps my experience (and kundalini awakening experience in general) signifies a quantum leap to new movements of vital energy. In other words, kundalini awakening is the quantum leap of vital creativity.

We have discussed aspects of vital creativity before in connection with the guna of tejas and the pitta dosha in connection with the navel chakra and the heart. Traditional kundalini awakening includes the brow chakra in the equation. Under the guidance of quantum science, we now can include more of the brain chakras in the kundalini awakening equation.

Why is this important? Aging, as conventional researchers have argued, involves the "normal" reduction of the functions of the organs at the various chakras. Since in quantum science the physiology is not fixed, if the chakra can be opened, the organs at a chakra can behave in a more quantum coherent way, and this reduces or may even eliminate the deterioration. In this way, for people who let the opportunity for a transition pass in response to the call of holotropy, we suggest the following recourse to achieve a continuing quality of life and death with dignity:

1. To develop a belief system overhaul beginning with a thorough understanding of the meaning and purpose of life and death, in particular, the idea of reincarnation.
2. To develop a new perspective of aging, especially the conviction that quality of life is more important than quantity. This consists of examining how aging leads to reduced ability to get the juice of life from the existing physiology, and how an effort to opt for better physiology is worth it.
3. To engage in practices toward a better physiology. This results in the general development of positive emotional brain circuits. This is the key to quality of life via the elimination of emotional stress and the accentuation of a positive psychological bend.

Item No. 1 has been covered throughout this book, so no further discussion is necessary except to remind ourselves that to look at death as a passageway to the next life—as Tibetan researchers discovered centuries ago—eliminates a major component of fear and aversion to risk-taking that comes with aging: namely, the fear of death. An understanding of reincarnation also gives you an important new perspective: When you die, your material possessions don't go with you; what accompanies you is your karma—your character traits and habit patterns of karma, your learned propensities. When you realize this, your later life becomes a preparation for the next and this gives you motivation to develop new habits to make healthy software for the reentry to a life of meaning and purpose, archetypes.

Some karma-comeuppance will happen for your past indiscretions, no doubt, including severe chronic diseases such as cancer, heart disease, or arthritis. But one thing you can be certain of: You do not have to fear Alzheimer's and the like. Death with dignity is assured.

THEORY OF AGING

There are numerous theories addressing aging, but they generally fall into two main categories: aging as a programmed state and aging resulting from an accumulation of damage.

The programmed death is part of the software of every living cell. The researcher Leonard Hayflick discovered what is now called the Hayflick Effect. A cell can only divide some fifty times or so. With each division of the cell, the cell cap called telomere shortens; after fifty or so divisions, it disappears entirely, and the cell dies. This genetic software also suggests on the average human life span should extend no more than a hundred years or so.

Some aging researchers emphasize that aging is more a deterioration of survival programs of physiology rather than a programmed part of individual cell-development. On the face of it, if the software is complex as it is for higher animals, the software is going to be distributed over many individual cells; if a cell crucial to a part of the complex software dies, the function will be compromised. Additionally, there will be cellular environmental factors: accumulation of oxidant, disruption of regulatory pathways from the hypothalamus and pituitary to the other glands crucial for organ functioning, etc.

There are, of course, repair mechanisms: regeneration. There are stem cells and the liturgical potentiality should be available to freshly program some of them to repair the lost complexity. But the issue is more complex than that. Stem cells also die; they too are subject to the Hayflick Effect. Besides, according to quantum science, there is that question of will to live that activates the body wisdom. It is a fact that, as we get old, our injuries take longer to heal. It could be partly due to an overall reduction of the zing to survive.

It is safe to conclude that this buildup of software damage amplified by the decreased capacity to repair mechanism is affected by programmed senescence—the Hayflick Effect. So the complex interplay of environment and genetic predisposition may result in aging. In other words, programmed cell death and aging as a result of cellular damage are not mutually exclusive and both together address the why and how of aging.

The remedy of quantum integral medicine should now be obvious. We employ quantum yoga techniques of software maintenance along with techniques of quantum healing (to activate the repair mechanism) in addition to the nutrition programs of Ayurveda and naturopathy—herbs and food supplements.

For more adventurous people, there is also soul-making and the possibility of even more advanced physiology.

Below, we examine some details of individual organ function deterioration and try to evaluate the efficacy of a QIM health management program for all the important organ groups.

ORGAN FUNCTION DETERIORATION WITH AGING

According to gerontologist G. E. Taffet, "General aging changes in the body are related to loss of complexity in physiologic function such as cardiac, neurologic, and stress response." With cell death, when there are fewer quantum potentialities to maintain homeostasis available, a phenomenon called homeo-stenosis takes place. *Stenosis* is a generic medical word used to denote the narrowing of a passageway.

Body mechanisms such as the Circadian rhythm of maintenance of body temperature, the accumulation of the stress cortisol in plasma, and secretion of melatonin by the pineal gland and sleep, are all affected due to general lack of situational creativity—vital vayu. This lack of vital creativity for making minor adjustments of the software is responsible for a general inflexibility of the system to effect minor changes in response to the need of the moment. Lack of vital creativity of vayu leads to the accumulation of the dosha of vata at the physical level so much so that in Indian culture, it is still customary for people to refer to old-age health problems generally as, "I have vata."

So, aging cannot be corrected by automatic situational adjustments, that is the whole point. The body's so-called wisdom, the conditioned spectrum of potentialities that vayu works with, is no longer doing the job, and tejas—fundamental creativity needs to be invoked.

Conventionalists prescribe physical exercise and mental agility. Recent data is showing that doing these things in groups (thus bringing nonlocality in action) works even better, but even that is not enough. You need to add quantum Ayurvedic and yogic remedies. Even traditional Ayurveda makes one very important point here: The overall homeo-stenosis that we call part of aging is also due to an accumulation of toxins—ama in Sanskrit—due to kapha dosha. The cleaning of the toxin accumulation is achieved by pancha karma—a five-fold cleaning ritual discussed earlier. To this, when you add a combination of Ayurvedic herbs and vital exercises, quantum style, you've got it.

A brief reminder: We call the vital exercises done in the quantum style "quantum yoga." How is it different? In ordinary yoga, there are two prevalent styles—fast yoga and slow yoga. Fast yoga is hardly more than physical stretching exercises—do-do-do. Slow yoga, on the other hand, when we pay attention to vital movements, is an attempt to make yoga asana practice into a do-be-do-be-do style of vital exercise; but let's face it, do-do-do still dominates. If, on the other hand, when we do yoga stretching like animals do, that is, maintain a posture over some time, it is the vital equivalent of be-be-be. Doing these two styles in tandem produces the do-be-do-be-do process of perfection for creativity. Of course, this results in an occasional quantum leap of vital energy, a mini kundalini awakening that can restore body's healing wisdom back.

This restores the system as follows: As the system quantum jumps to higher functioning, the organs function at an elevated level. Some of the organs get needed rest while others function in more of a quantum coherent mode. In that mode, new creative potentialities can be actualized to program a stem cell for the regeneration of the missing part of the complex physiology.

If we have to practice quantum yoga for all of the physical systems going wrong simultaneously, the practice would be foreboding.

Fortunately, except for a few geriatric syndromes such as chronic fatigue and multiple sclerosis our physiology deteriorates system by system depending on your particular lifestyle. In previous chapters, we have discussed some of the lifestyle deterioration of the organs of the navel and the heart chakra—the gastro-intestinal and cardio-vascular and immune systems, respectively. Here, we will take up the case of a few more.

For the cardiovascular system, let's talk about one thing though: the hardening of artery walls and stiffening of the veins. Lethargic vitality (kapha dosha) leads to ama accumulation everywhere when inertia generally prevails. Timely action of vayu keeps the problem at bay. In old age, excess vata becomes the order of the day, vayu is inoperable, and, due to the accumulated ama (molecules of inflammation and cholesterol), the arteries harden and the veins stiffen, resulting in hypertension.

High blood pressure is such a dangerous condition to carry in old age (because it increases the chance of heart attack and stroke) that we prescribe not only Ayurvedic remedies (herbs), naturopathic remedies (food and natural supplements), and quantum yoga exercises but also allopathic remedies such as blood-pressure medicine.

AGING AND THE ELIMINATION SYSTEM

Let's take up some of the aging changes that occur in the elimination system mainly due to changes in smooth muscle activity and the body's absorption of nutrients from food intake:

1. A decrease in the production of saliva
2. Desynchronization of contraction and relaxation of smooth muscle movement affecting sphincter control, making swallowing less effective
3. Altered metabolism of proteins and absorption of nutrients

4. Prolonged transit time for feces movement
5. Atrophy of gastrointestinal mucosa, the ama
6. Decreased strength of colonic muscles
7. Decrease in liver and pancreas size

Item 1 leads to loss of appetite. According to Ayurveda, this is due to an imbalance of the various tastes: We need to satisfy all of our six tastes: sweet, sour, salty, bitter, pungent, and astringent. The Ayurvedic remedy is *rasayana*—healing through balancing our diet to include all six tastes. This involves consciously correcting the preference you have developed because of dosha aggravation.

Generally speaking, with aggravated vata and kapha, we prefer sweet, sour, salty, and bitter, and the astringent and pungent tastes promote tejas, which is precisely what rasayana prescribes as part of the remedy.

Items 2 to 6 all contribute to constipation. Here again, panchakarma helps, as does food with adequate fiber. When this is not enough, Ayurvedic herbs are more effective than traditional allopathic laxatives. All of this is only a temporary cure, however.

To make a lasting remedy, we have to recourse to quantum yoga—vital and mental creativity, in this case, because the negative emotion of fear enters the picture in a major way.

Transforming fear into courage is basic to all applications of quantum yoga for the quality control of old age. Here, the mental component is the wrong belief system; we already have addressed that.

Item 7 is a navel chakra concern and requires quantum yoga exercises and fundamental creativity for regeneration using stem cells.

AGING OF THE NAVEL CHAKRA ORGANS: METABOLISM AND VISCERAL FAT IN OLD AGE

There is a widespread belief that metabolism decreases progressively at old age and many old-age problems such as obesity and Type II diabetes happen mainly due to this. But this belief needs to change radically—and, thankfully, it is. Recent clinical data has established that metabolism drastically changes at the age of fifteen months, decreasing from a very high rate to about half that rate, and then at about age sixty, it begins decreasing progressively. Between the ages of about twenty to sixty, the metabolic rate remains roughly constant, though the exact amount varies from person to person. In other words, there is a lot of heterogeneity for the metabolic rate, a fact that supports the Ayurvedic dosha theory of heterogeneity.

But what is most important to note is this: The (physical) energy spent toward metabolism by people who do regular exercise goes toward muscle-building whereas, for sedentary people, the energy goes to do-do-do maintenance activities and—guess what?—toward emotional stress response, immune inflammation, and visceral fat. It is the latter that leads to navel-chakra organ disfunction. Visceral fat is the abdominal fat that accumulates in the abdominal cavity, producing what's known as a "beer belly." This happens mainly in men, and contrasts with all other fat, such as subcutaneous fat or women's fat in thighs, hips, and buttocks.

Some visceral fat acts as an extra emergency reservoir of physical energy. However, while excessive visceral fat covers the navel organs such as the liver, stomach, and pancreas, along with the spaces in between these organs, the fat impacts their activity, producing malfunction.

One way that the malfunction works is what is called the metabolic syndrome—insulin resistance, or the loss of the cell's sensitivity to insulin. The muscle cells surrounding the pancreas in a normal situation soaks up the insulin, which enables the absorption of sugar, especially glucose from the bloodstream. Under insulin resistance, these cells do not absorb the sugar in the bloodstream, and thus they produce the high blood sugar symptomatic of Type II diabetes.

During middle age, quantum yoga can help prevent visceral fat and metabolic syndrome. Unbalanced ojas—inertia—is what allows the accumulation of excess abdominal fat. Yoga activates vital creativity—vayu—and keeps the systems in balance. Most importantly, by activating tejas as necessary, quantum yoga can elevate the physiology by reprogramming the stem cells with normal sensitivity to insulin and absorbing the excess sugar from the bloodstream.

Though the metabolic rate remains the same as we go through adulthood and middle age, most sedentary people begin to develop a beer belly and weight gain (obesity) during middle age, and this remains a problem ever after, if it is not properly addressed. The consensus on developing obesity is that it must be due to minor causes like genetic predisposition and hormonal changes as well as major factors like stressful lifestyle and eating habits—eating what, how, and when we want to. Many people who develop obesity are under emotional stress and eat processed fast food in a hurry, not just when they are hungry but also when they are stressed.

AGING OF THE HEART-CHAKRA ORGANS

As for aging effects on heart-chakra organs, the phenomenon of thymic involution—the reduction of the size of the thymus gland—needs to be considered. Thymic involution may affect our ability to suspend thymus activity later in life, making the quantum leap required for love more difficult to achieve. From a quantum-science standpoint, this is one issue that everyone should address before age sixty when thymus involution seriously sets in.

In other words, if you continue the "iron-man syndrome" into your old age, you will be more vulnerable to immune system disorders, including impaired autoimmune response and much of quantum science will have lost its potency for you.

In the same vein, another old-age effect is the reduction of red bone marrow, which are the stem cells for both red blood cells and white blood cells. This is bad news because fundamental creativity at the heart chakra may require stem cells for regeneration.

AGING CHANGES IN THE ENDOCRINE SYSTEM: CREATIVITY AT THE MIDBRAIN CHAKRA

The effects of aging on the glands produce some atrophy and decrease hormonal secretion. Changes in hormonal action may be the most apparent change in aging. These changes in function are most spectacular in insulin production and glucose-level maintenance; the malfunction here is responsible for Type II diabetes.

The excretion of feces prevents accumulation of excess vata and its aggravation; similarly, the excretion of urine gets rid of excess pitta—gastric ama. Both these functions are affected by changes in adrenal gland—the origin of stress hormones.

Let's focus next on the pancreas, which controls insulin production to maintain the blood's glucose level. The relationship of the pancreas and stomach (plus the liver and gallbladder) is similar to the relationship of the thymus and the heart, except it is reversed. When we fast, giving the stomach rest, the pancreas becomes more quantum and coherent in its rhythm, and insulin production, likewise, is better regulated. This prevents both hyper- and hypoglycemia, both major factors of Type II diabetes.

Perspiration—the product of the sweat glands—is one of the ways that excess kapha accumulations are eliminated from the body. So here is another red flag to watch at old age: Are you sweating enough?

The thyroid gland controls the metabolic rate of the body. Aging often produces hypothyroidism. Thyroid health depends on adequate iodine intake and is easy to maintain. Pay attention to your diet for adequate iodine whenever you notice the symptoms of hypothyroidism such as fatigue, increased sensitivity to cold, puffy face, etc.

The pituitary gland is the master gland and is, in turn, controlled by the hypothalamus, a midbrain gland that is notable for producing the love hormone oxytocin. The main function of the hypothalamus is to maintain homeostasis of the body, which it does mainly by controlling the pituitary gland. The hypothalamus is the key: Quantum science suggests a novel way for you to gain conscious control over the entire glandular system, including the endocrine glands.

Previously, we focused on the brain takeovers of the body chakras. In quantum science, the brain can only give potentiality for consciousness to choose from. To produce any software, we need conscious awareness—a self-identity—to collapse experience and make memory. Since the brain takeover begins in mammals with the development of the midbrain, we must postulate that mammals have a midbrain chakra and a self-identity associated with it that is active in the first year of babyhood and becomes unconscious with the gradual development of the cortical self after the first year of babyhood. This is how we lose conscious control of the functions of the midbrain consisting of the administration of negative emotional and pleasure circuits and the hypothalamus.

How do we regain control? The idea of using vital creativity and kundalini awakening suggests itself. Can we do this? There is evidence in the spiritual literature of kundalini masters, who have such emotional equanimity that it could only come from the awakening of the midbrain self-identity and a restoration of conscious control over the midbrain organs' software.

The do-be-do-be-do practices of quantum yoga and chi gong should be adequate for the awakening of the midbrain chakra. Of course, the design of quantum yoga specific to the midbrain chakra will take some trial and error and concerted effort, which is under research.

There is also a practice in Taoist medicine that can be useful here. The blocked vital energy at the low chakras—*jing*—is to be raised or transformed into *shen*—the vital energy of the awakened midbrain chakra. We do it by repeated visualization of light gradually illuminating the body starting from the low chakras and rising all the way to the midbrain.

There are challenges against this kind of practice when old age sets in because of overall decline in brain mass. A reduction of brain's response to hormone activity occurs with aging, which affects both brain and body-wide functioning. Take note of this and begin your practices at your midlife.

THE AGING OF THE NEURONAL SYSTEM AND THE CORTEX: ORGANS OF THE BROW CHAKRA

Aging of the cortex and the neurological system consists of a 30 percent loss of brain mass, including gray matter, by age eighty. Undoubtedly, this will produce an overall decline in the production of neurotransmitters, some memory loss, and a reduction of response to both external and internal stimuli, etc.

The main brain health concern today is dementia, especially Alzheimer's disease. Alzheimer's researchers talk about a mysterious process of inflammation and try to explain it in vaguely material terms. But the truth is, nobody knows why Alzheimer's occurs. Perhaps allopathic medicine's understanding of Alzheimer's disease will evolve the same way understanding of cholesterol has.

Let us explain. Decades ago, the allopathic belief was that it is cholesterol accumulation that you have to watch out for when it comes to preventing coronary heart attacks. Allopathic physicians have quietly undergone a complete shift in their attitude toward cholesterol after many experts began to point out the fallacy of making the molecule of cholesterol that the body itself makes aplenty the culprit of coronary artery blockage. Gradually, after repeated clinical studies, it was finally concluded that the cholesterol blockage of arteries is not a cause of the blockage but is both a trigger and an effect of the inflammation that is the actual cause of arterial blockage. But what is inflammation?

Researchers have not made the same mistake when it comes to Alzheimer's; they do not say that amyloid protein is the cause of Alzheimer's. They correctly point to inflammation as the cause. But then again, what is inflammation and what produces it?

Materially speaking, the inflammation consists of inflammatory molecules produced by a malfunctioning overactive immune system. But what causes the immune system malfunction? If you ask an Ayurvedic expert about such things as coronary blockage and amyloid plaques that cover memory-neurons, the expert will blanketly blame everything as the effects of a lifestyle causing a vata dosha. Initially, when I (Amit) first heard that, I did not pay attention. Vata dosha is not specific enough to be helpful, or so I thought.

But my unconscious processing after some conscious deliberation led to a new idea. Perhaps inflammation is not physical in how it is initiated at all, but rather is initiated by a vital phenomenon such as vata aggravation, or more accurately, both vata and kapha aggravation, the yin-yang imbalance.

Here is how yin-yang imbalance works: It is a lifestyle propensity—the vital equivalent of a mind-brain dosha of mental hyperactivity. In mental hyperactivity, the mind moves in a fickle way from one thing to another, so when a real situation arises, the mind cannot focus or apply its quality of rajas (the ability to engage situational creativity) to creatively solve the problem. In inflammation, the vital-physical has picked up the habit of easy distraction and cannot be brought to focus when needed.

Like the inflammation of the arteries, the inflammation of the memory neurons is the product of immune malfunction due to loneliness and lack of love in an elderly person's life. The neurons are organs; normally, they have their V-organs run by inertia—ojas. Kapha accumulation—stagnant vitality—produces ama, the amyloid beta, at the inflammation sites; normally, another mechanism—vayu, vital creativity—operates to clean up the ama. With inflammatory molecules at the site, vital creativity cannot engage and the ameloid beta (or cholesterol for the arteries) goes on accumulating.

Simply put, due to vata aggravation, the patient's body-wisdom has difficulty making the vital creative adjustments to the vital software to activate the proteins needed to clean up the mess, producing dementia.

What produces this kapha-vata aggravation? It is a lifestyle issue. Information processing produces mental hyperactivity which, in turn, produces vital hyperactivity in the brain memory neurons' vital software. In this way, our modern lifestyle of constant information processing may be predisposing young people to future Alzheimer's. Excessive information-processing individuals are also at greater risk of cognitive decline in general with age. Such aging changes may include:

- Reduction of the production of neurotransmitters such as serotonin and acetylcholine, which may cause sleep disorders.
- Reduction of sites for the uptake of dopamine as well as dopamine transporters will reduce the positive feelings of eating and sexual pleasure.
- Depletion of the binding sites of the neurotransmitter GABA—gamma-aminobutyric acid.
- Decreased quantity of nerve fibers of the motor, sensory, and autonomic nervous systems. This reduces an elderly person's ability for sensory processing and response.
- Decrease of the conduction velocity of electrical signals through the nerves. This may affect our intuitive facility, which requires quantum self-identity involving the coherent quantum participation of the many organs of the brain simultaneously.
- Decline of signal transduction rate between brainstem and spinal cord.
- Muscular atrophy—general deterioration of muscle activity.
- Weakening of heart-rate response to arterial blood pressure changes.

Let's emphasize that magic cure allopathic drugs for either Alzheimer's or general cognitive decline may never be found. Prevention is one solution involving brain-mind-vital exercises, quantum-style. An even better solution may involve the crown chakra. The main crown chakra organ is the parietal lobe, which makes a homuncular image of our entire body organs so that it can be used for monitoring the body. In this way, the parietal lobe is responsible for overall body identity and yet its experiences, which require a separate self-identity, are unconscious in us.

What happens if we can have conscious control over the parietal lobe? That is, if we can awaken a self-identity there; after all, it has all the tangled hierarchical necessities. An awakened healthy crown chakra may be all we need to prevent all cognitive decline.

GERIATRIC SYNDROMES

Certain health conditions, called geriatric syndromes, occur more often in the elderly. These conditions often lead to morbidity and poor outcomes for healing in aging patients with chronic diseases. The list consists of:

- general skin breakout
- changes in sleep pattern
- gait disorders such as frequent falls
- sensory deficits such as hearing loss
- weight loss and nutrient imbalances
- fatigue
- dizziness
- frailty
- delirium

From a quantum-science point of view, these syndromes act as warning: They are indicative of the need for urgent attention to holistic healthcare. Our preliminary studies indicate that the quantum integrative medicine approach, when instituted, eliminates these symptoms almost immediately.

OLD PEOPLE AND ILLNESS: FLU AND COVID 19

To young people, a virus is a nuisance—a suffering-producing nuisance, to be sure, but no more than that. To old people, even a flu infection is a crisis. And if it is the current coronavirus, Covid 19, it is a downright life-threatening crisis.

Quantum science says we experience fear and anxiety in our psyche. Objects in the psyche are quantum objects. In contrast with Newtonian physics, which is deterministic, inflexible, and unchangeable, quantum physics is the physics of possibility. When you behave from conditioned homeostasis, your psyche becomes Newtonian too, making you the prey of built-in negativity. It is up to you—up to all of us—to choose to stay with conditioned and Newtonian homeostasis of the psyche or opt for the quantum approach. Yes, quantum science says, you can say no to conditioning. If you intend to choose new possibilities, higher consciousness will hear you if your intention is synchronized with the purposive movements of consciousness, and if it does, you get to manifest your wish.

There are both physical and mental aspects of our problem with the coronavirus. The physical aspect is to find preventive measures: What possibilities can we choose to keep us physically healthy at this time when the corona virus is spreading exponentially—that is, apart from the obvious hygienic measures, of which isolation is the most effective choice but gives us mental anxiety arising from the disruption of our regular normal functional routine?

PHYSICAL ASPECTS OF COVID 19

Let's consider Covid 19's physical aspects first. What's a virus? How do viruses work? In quantum physics, we distinguish between the living and the nonliving. Only the living can be conscious, can live, can experience. The nonliving exists in the unconscious, and unless a sentient being experiences it, the nonliving has no manifest existence.

QUANTUM GERONTOLOGY

A virus is a half-alive structure; though nonliving, it is a strand of potentially replicable nucleic acid molecule in potentiality. It cannot replicate, but it needs proteins from a host to help make its own proteins, and then it can reproduce, living and rapidly multiplying in the host's suitable organs. If the organs are not functioning properly, it can defeat the organs' defence mechanism, the immune system.

We hear a lot about strengthening the immune system from our allopathic medical experts. They have no theory of what makes the immune system and other organs function, but they have learned a lot from empirical data. On that basis, they tell us about food that can help us: ginger, onion, garlic, turmeric, oranges, and the like, all of which is good.

However, can we do better now that we have a science of the living software, the vital body, in quantum science? Organs have a molecular physical hardware which is governed by physical laws. But living software is purposive and physical laws are casual; purposive laws govern the subtle bodies of the psyche because they are nonphysical. These quantum software laws of the vital are telling us a lot of new things, the most important of which is the science behind the chakras. We have to learn to use this new science.

The immune system straddles the heart and the navel chakra. At the heart is the crucial thymus gland, which distinguishes between the body molecules and foreign molecules and kills off the foreign molecules. The immune system is our defence system.

But this a prosaic, material way of thinking about the immune function. The conscious way to think about it is that the thymus gland distinguishes between "me" and "not-me." It works like this: I see you; you are not-me to me, and my body's immune system will defend me against you. But if I love you, I include you in what I feel as me. What has happened? My immune system has been put in momentary suspension.

For its well-being, the immune system needs this continual suspension because it provides it with rest just like the neocortex. Wherever there is a self to experience, there is a need for rest. There are only three chakras with which we have this experience: the neocortex, the heart, and the navel. All of the organs at these chakras need rest.

Back to the coronavirus. One of its preferred hosts is a malfunctioning lung, another one are the blood vessels. Malfunctioning implies that the hardware-software, physical-vital connection has gone awry. If the lungs (or the bold vessels) are healthy, the virus does not get its preferred host, and its effect will be mild.

So, here is our first quantum preventive healing hint for how to improve the vital software of the lungs and/or the blood vessels. One immediate remedy is this: breathe, breathe, breathe. Oxygen is deadly for the virus.

But of course, if the immune system is healthy, it will succeed in killing off such a mild attack. Even if the lungs (and the blood vessels) are not so great, but the immune system is healthy, there will be complications, but sooner or later the immune system will succeed; it is only a matter of time. The patient survives.

The fatal situation is that when the lungs and the blood circulation system are not healthy, neither is the immune system. Then, when its weak response is not helping the lungs, it goes berserk, over-functioning, going into overdrive, and it is the overdriven immune system reactions that eventually kills the body.

So, our second quantum preventive healing hint is this: The way to keep the immune system from malfunctioning is to give it needed rest.

There is another interesting symptom of coronavirus—fatigue all over the body, which I have already noted is due to the general disconnect of the living hardware and software. This is an indication that coronavirus has actually intruded into all of the organs in the body.

So, our third quantum healing hint is this: Keep all your vital software in dynamic balance. Be creative about caring for your vital body, all of it. (See Chapter 13.)

MENTAL/EMOTIONAL ASPECTS OF COVID 19

Not surprisingly, the emotional aspects of dealing with the coronavirus epidemic arise from the breakdown of our daily routine; moreover, most of us are busy do-do-do people, and we are not used to being with ourselves. Our moods swing often, even at work. But business and the culture of emotion suppression prevail. Alone with ourselves, even with our job to do at home, the mood swings haunt us, and actually we raid the refrigerator more often so we can keep anxieties at bay. We are suffering from what my friend, filmmaker Carl Blake, calls *abusity*. People who have child abuse in their developmental history and traumatic memory, as a result, have a tendency of overeating and getting obese. Those tendencies can come back in a hurry during middle and old age.

Others have relationship problems. Today's people never learn or have the opportunity to learn about relationships, especially intimate relationships. It all happens on the job for most people.

Many people who live alone suffer from loneliness. This is because they have never learned to love themselves. Also, what is there to love if their psyches are full of emotional garbage in a culture which does not teach them emotional hygiene?

Some of the mental/emotional issues are the same as the physical-vital: how to institute proper hygiene of your brain, organ physiology, and maintain healthy vital software. Additional issues include how to maintain a healthy immune system and how to prevent its tendency of excessive defensiveness due to preoccupation with lower survival needs. The quantum remedy is to switch to focusing on higher-level needs such as how to love your partner and also yourself. These issues have already been discussed in earlier chapters (see especially Chapters 9 and 12). In this way, if you follow a quantum lifestyle and learn the lessons of quantum integrative medicine, you can overcome health challenges, even in your old age.

How do you strengthen a weak pair of lungs (and blood circulation too)? The do-be-do-be-do practice involving the breathing practice pranayama works miracles to strengthen the lungs and, in fact, all the organs. It consists of alternative deep inhaling: The organs burst into function, one by one, as you inhale and supply oxygen to the organs in your abdomen, chest, and throat. This is the *do* phase. Then you deliberately hold your breath for a few seconds. This is called *kumbhaka* in Sanskrit, but you can easily recognize it as the *be* phase of the creative process. And then you exhale slowly, so that deoxygenation occurs as the organ progressively stops functioning, halting the movement of vital energy. Repeat this a few times.

Notice that the lungs straddle the heart chakra and the throat chakra. The throat chakra function is expression—speech, singing, etc. Speech involves the tongue, which is also a speech organ, and is the reason why many Covid victims suffer a loss of taste. A very good practice for strengthening the throat chakra is singing in the shower—the tiles reflect the sound, producing reverberation, and your singing sounds inspirational, even to yourself.

PSYCHIATRY'S DARKEST ASPECTS IN THE BIG PHARMA MONOPOLY

Why has there been such a dramatic rise in mental disease and invariably increased use of prescribed psychiatric drugs in recent years? Could it simply be because more people are getting mentally disabled? Or could it be due to a number of other dark and sinister aspects at work related to psychiatry's connection to Big Pharma's profit machine? In light of this question, here are some of psychiatry's darkest aspects in the Big Pharma monopoly.

CHEMICAL IMBALANCE THEORY: A BIG PHARMA SCANDAL?

Big Pharma has made trillions of dollars in psychiatric drug sales on the chemical imbalance theory, much of it from older people. The widely accepted principle of chemical imbalance is based on the idea that mental diseases like depression (from which many elderly people suffer) are caused by an imbalance of chemical neurotransmitters such as dopamine in the brain. However, there is no scientific evidence to support this theory. For example, there is no evidence proving that the accepted cause of depression is an imbalance of the neurotransmitter serotonin.

Although rigorously promoted by Big Pharma, many psychiatrists, and sales and marketing representatives, the portfolio-expanding money-spinning pharmaceutical drug treatment model of mental disease is based on much fiction. With the baseless chemical imbalance theory, the tragedy is that patients are never healed although some drugs bring the symptoms down to tolerable levels. As patients continue to suffer, we must ask: What about the dangerous side effects of these drugs, especially for the elderly?

On the encouraging side, research suggests that immune imbalances rather than faulty neurochemistry are the causes of severe mental disease such as clinical depression. The good news is that some researchers are switching to an immune inflammation theory of psychosis. In that case, quantum science's answer is simply a healthy immune system, an awakening of the heart, etc., as preventive medicine. If prevention fails, a patient has to try quantum healing of both vital and mental to bring back meaning and purpose in life because the lack of meaning and purpose is the root cause of psychosis, especially depression.

In summary, let us just say that quantum integrative medicine covers much more ground than the usual holistic framework in both disease prevention and healing for the elderly. It is literally equivalent to the positive mental health program of transpersonal psychology that Abraham Maslow initiated.

The best option for any person is to respond positively to holotropy at midlife whenever the drive hits, and then enter a creative quantum lifestyle of soul-making in order to achieve both health and happiness. This is the true holistic health practice.

chapter seventeen

PREVENTIVE MEDICINE LESSON 7: HOLISTIC HEALTH, QUANTUM STYLE

The poet John Keats famously wrote to a friend, "Call the world, if you please, / 'The Vale of soul-making.'" This, according to quantum science, is the essential purpose of the human life. If we serve this purpose, the world would indeed be a better place to live for the coming generations.

First of all, let's talk about the concept of soul. Confusion arises because we also use the word "soul" to denote the "me" that survives after death and takes rebirth. Can the two uses denote the same thing? Yes, they could, but realistically, for 85 percent of people today, they probably don't. Let's try to understand why.

The soul is also a station we posit in the so-called great chain of being: body, mind, soul, spirit. In this usage, the ego is one with the ordinary body physiology that we are born with; likewise, the mind, which remains in the domain of what is known. The soul is a station of conscious awareness beyond ego; there is a progression of such stations. Spirit, of course, refers to the quantum self.

On the way, the soul is a station reached by delving and embodying what is unknown—both vital and mental. There is also the trivial unknown of the imagination. Not that. The unknown here is arrived at by changing the contexts of feeling and thinking to the archetypes. It takes creativity and quantum leaps.

For the vital, it takes tejas—the capacity for fundamental vital creativity—and for the mental, it takes sattva—fundamental mental creativity—to discover a new archetypal context. This is what the challenge of soul-making consists of.

Archetypes bring purpose to your life. The mind, when elevated by the archetypes, brings meaning back; it sees the feelings generated by the archetypal elevation as positive. Together with archetypal exploration, you can develop positive emotions and you can make positive emotional brain circuits involving the body's chakra as well as the brain's. These positive emotions are the key to the elevated living of the soul—in expansion of consciousness.

The expansion of consciousness is experienced as happiness. In this way, not only are you having the soul-level of positive health we have already discussed but also positive mental health. What's the point? Happiness brings you the much-needed motivation for the soul journey. That and the drive of holotropy, which is strong in midlife.

The steps you take along the journey of happiness is an important subject by itself and is presented in Amit's book *Quantum Psychology and the Science of Happiness*, written in collaboration with psychologist Sunita Pattani.

The journey of happiness gives us soul software but not the ability to use the software as and when needed, appropriately, and without effort. This ability is intelligence and this is what we need for having a soul-identity. How to develop intelligence, especially archetypal or supramental intelligence, is beyond the scope of this book.

It takes major changes in your belief system—primacy of consciousness instead of primacy of matter, the nonphysical nature of feelings and thinking, intuitions and archetypes, and real creativity. The most radical of the belief system change for a Westerner is reincarnation.

REINCARNATION: DEVELOPING A HEALTHY PERSPECTIVE FOR DEATH AND DYING

If one asks for that one cause that drives healthcare costs in America up and up and up, it would be, according to many people, the money we spend to keep people alive in the last three months of their lives. Death is not only regarded as painful and undesirable, but essentially as an encounter with the great void, nothingness, a finale. And that is the source of the fear of death.

But a science within the primacy of consciousness tells us otherwise very quickly. Consciousness is the ground of being—it never dies. Additionally, we have the subtle bodies, the mental and the vital of which the personality arises from conditioning. When we look at the mental and vital conditioning, we find that this is the result of modification of the mathematics, the algorithms that determine the probabilities associated with quantum possibilities. The "quantum" memory of these modifications is not written anywhere locally, so it can survive the local existence in one space-time to another, giving us the phenomenon popularly called reincarnation. What survives, then, are not bodies, but propensities of using the mind and the vital body, propensities that are popularly called karma.

But why do we reincarnate? Because it takes time to awaken soul and supramental intelligence. It requires many permutations and combinations of vital and mental patterns (which Easterners call karma) and many quantum leaps to eventually learn the contexts that constitute supramental intelligence.

So, what is death, according to this perspective? Death is an important part of the learning journey that we are on. Death is a prolonged period of unconscious processing, the second-most important stage of creativity. The evidence of this is found in near-death experiences.

Near-death experiences have been known for some time. Some people who can be regarded as clinically dead, for example, due to a cardiac arrest, after being resuscitated, report numinous experiences—being out of the body, meeting a spiritual master, going through a tunnel, etc. How do we explain such experiences that require a subject-object split, when a person is clinically dead? The explanation is unconscious processing and collapse by delayed choice. The near-death subjects were processing possibilities unconsciously while dead; only after they were revived did their possibility waves collapse, and their experience took place retroactively. This retroactive collapse of an entire pathway of events leading to the current event is called delayed choice in physics. It follows that if the patient were not revived, he or she would have continued unconscious processing until the next birth. And the unconscious that is processed is mainly the collective unconscious, quite useful for creativity.

DISEASE AS OPPORTUNITY

We previously mentioned that many mind-body healers think that disease is the creation of the patient. "What do you gain by creating your disease?" is their favorite question for their patient. This kind of question only confuses the patient and makes them feel guilty.

And yet, the mind-body healer is seeing an opportunity here that the patient needs to see if he or she is ready for it. The correct question is, "Now that you have the disease, instead of giving it a negative meaning, can you give a positive meaning to it? Suppose you take the responsibility for the disease and ask, 'Why did I create this disease for myself? What do I want to learn from it?'"

A disease is an expression of enormous incongruence. In a physical injury, for example, the hardware of the injured organ becomes incongruent with its software; this negates the feeling of vitality at that organ, a feeling of lack of vitality that we experience as illness. If the disease originates at the mental level because of the mentalization of a feeling, the incongruence will be experienced at all levels—mental, vital, and physical. We think something, we feel something else, and physical body acts in still another way.

How do we reestablish congruence so that the mind, the vital energies, and the physical representations act in congruence? The answer, in a nutshell, is: supramental intelligence. A mind-body disease is a fantastic opportunity, a very loud wakeup call to awaken our supramental intelligence—*buddhi* in Sanskrit. The ancient seers of India knew about supramental intelligence.

When we engage in supramental intelligence in the acts of creativity, we can use a quantum leap of creative insight to the service of outer creativity, or we can use it to explore ourselves, in inner creativity. In the same way, if we are only interested in supramental intelligence to heal our disease, it is like engaging in outer creativity. Good, but we are limiting the application. It is entirely possible to use supramental intelligence gained in quantum healing in further creative exploration of the mental/vital/physical domain with the objective of spiritual growth. Then, it is inner creativity, and it is great. We recommend you read the physician Bernie Siegel's book *Peace, Love & Healing* for many anecdotes about exceptional people who followed this path from disease to healing to inner wholeness.

SUPRAMENTAL INTELLIGENCE

Health and happiness require an elevated level of being in which the loss of complex software that comes with aging is more than made up by the availability of new potentialities to make new better software. If you start soul-making at midlife, there is no need to worry about the availability of stem cells for regeneration.

However, there is another important step here. You have made software, but you have not changed. You are still in your ego. You have to choose consciously the new positive emotional circuits to stay positive. In your unconscious moments, and there are always some, you may fall prey to old habits that can invite disease and unhappiness.

The remedy is to make a quantum leap in who you are, along with developing the new software. This crucial series of quantum leaps take you successively to higher and higher stations of the soul.

What are the characteristics of these stations? What do you have now that you did not have before? You have real intelligence, higher intelligence than the IQ that masquerades as intelligence today. Intelligence is the ability for appropriate action, appropriate to the needs of the moment. This is also a subject by itself and will be presented in our upcoming book *The Awakening of Intelligence*.

The highest rung of intelligence is supramental intelligence: It arrives from the exploration of the supramental archetypes culminating in the archetype of wholeness and an integration of all our dichotomies and conflicts.

In this way, the archetypal journey of exploration, of soul-making, ends up as a journey of the archetype of wholeness. In your training as a healer, this is the journey you have been on all the time. Now it is properly codified and scientized. We are convinced that this way of thinking about yourself and your exploration should help integrate your profession with your life.

AGELESS BODY, TIMELESS MIND

The title of the section is taken from the title of one of Deepak Chopra's books published in the 1990s, perhaps a bit ahead of its time. Later on, the development of quantum science shows that it is impossible to achieve a timeless mind because that would involve living in the present-centeredness of the quantum self in perpetuity. Our brain does not allow that. But how about an ageless body? How about immortality?

A great sage in Vedic India, Yajnabalkya, had enjoyed a teaching career after attaining enlightenment. Now he was ready to retire to the Himalayas. He asked his young wife, Maitreyi, who was also his disciple, if she wanted to give up all this comfort and accompany him. To his bequest, Maitreyi said these words:

Yenaham namrita shyam
Tenaham kim kuriyam

"What will not make me immortal, what will I do with that?" Saying that, she went with her husband to explore further stations of the soul and more supramental intelligence. But how can anyone not see the importance of the human quest for if not immortality but for an ageless body, living in health until we have the last breath?

We have mentioned recent studies which show that living a purposeful life does increase long life and in good order. Does supramental intelligence, in addition to giving us optimum physiology of organs, also work at the cellular level, change a cell's prescribed physiology codified by the Hayflick Effect? We don't know yet, but we coauthors both hope so.

BIBLIOGRAPHY

Achterberg, Jeanne. 1985. *Imagery in Healing: Shamanism and Modern Medicine*. Boston: Shambhala Publications.

Adams, Patch. The Gesundheit Institute. https://www.patchadams.org/.

Adams, Scott. 2018. s.v. "a dopamine hit— ." Dilbert syndicated daily comic strip dated March 27, 2018. https://dilbert.com/.

Ader, Robert. 1981. *Psychoneuroimmunology*. New York: Academic Press.

Aspect, Alain. 1976. "Proposed experiment to test the nonseparability of quantum mechanics." *Physical Review* D 14: 1944.

Barasch, Marc Ian. 1993. *The Healing Path: A Soul Approach to Illness*. New York: Tarcher/Putnam.

Bartlett, Zane. 2014. *Embryo Project Encyclopedia*, s.v. "Leonard Hayflick 1928– ." Phoenix: ASU (Arizona State University). http://embryo.asu.edu/handle/10776/8042.

Benson, Herbert (with Miriam Z. Klipper). 1975. *The Relaxation Response*. New York: William Morrow & Company.

Benson, Herbert (with Marg Stark). 1996. *Timeless Healing: The Power and Biology of Belief*. New York: Scribner.

Bessinger, Donivan. 2009. *Foundations of Noetic Medicine: Practicing the Medicine of the Mind*. North Charleston, SC: BookSurge Publishing.

Byrd, Randolph C. 1988. "Positive therapeutic effects of intercessory prayer in a coronary care unit population." *Southern Medical Journal* 81 (7): 826–29.

Chopra, Deepak. 1989. *Quantum Healing: Exploring the Frontiers of Mind/Body Medicine*. New York: Bantam-Doubleday.

Chopra, Deepak. 1993. *Ageless Body, Timeless Mind: The Quantum Alternative to Growing Old*. London: Random House.

Chopra, Deepak. 2000. *Perfect Health: Harness the Power of Ayurveda to Balance Mind and Body*. New York: Three Rivers Press.

Chopra, Deepak, Rupert Sheldrake, and Jill Purce. 2006. *Of Sound Mind & Body: Music & Vibrational Healing*. DVD and online-streaming video. Directed by Sound Healing, produced by Jeff Volk. San Francisco: Macromedia Publishing (DVD). Seattle, WA: Amazon Studios (Amazon Prime online streaming).

Cousins, Norman. 1979. *Anatomy of an Illness as Perceived by the Patient: Reflections on Healing and Regeneration*. New York: W. W. Norton.

Cousins, Norman. 1989. *Head First: the Biology of Hope*. New York: Dutton.

Dalai Lama Renaissance. 2009. Directed by Khashyar Darvish, featuring Dalai Lama, Harrison Ford, Michael Beckwith, Fred Alan Wolf, Amit Goswami, and others. DVD. Los Angeles: Wakan Films/funded by Wakan Foundation for the Arts. http://www.dalailamafilm.com/facts.html.

Dossey, Larry. 1992. *Meaning and Medicine: Lessons from a Doctor's Tales of Breakthrough and Healing*. New York: Bantam Books.

Dossey, Larry. 2001. *Healing Beyond the Body: Medicine and the Infinite Reach of the Mind*. Boston: Shambhala Publications.

Drouin, Paul. 2014. *Creative Integrative Medicine: A Medical Doctor's Journey Toward a New Vision of Healthcare*. New York: Balboa Press.

Emoto, Masaro. 2005. Translated by Horiko Hosoyamada. *The True Power of Water: Healing and Discovering Ourselves*. New York: Atria/Simon & Schuster.

Eigen, Manfred. 1996. *Steps towards Life: A Perspective on Evolution*. Oxford, UK: Oxford University Press.

Frawley, David. 1989. *Ayurvedic Healing: A Comprehensive Guide*. Salt Lake City, UT: Passage Press.

Frawley, David. 1999. *Yoga and Ayurveda: Self-Healing & Self-Realization*. Twin Lakes, WI: Lotus Press.

Freidman, Howard S., and Stephanie Booth-Kewley. (1987). "The 'disease-prone' personality. A meta-analytic view of the construct." *American Psychology* 42 (6): 539–55. doi: 10.1037//0003-066x42.6.539.

BIBLIOGRAPHY

Freund, Alexandra M., et al. (Participants in the workshop "Motivation and Healthy Aging" in Zurich, Switzerland, December 2019). 2021. "Motivation and Healthy Aging: A Heuristic Model." *Journal of Gerontology*: Series B 76, issue supplement 2 (October): S97–S104. https://doi.org/10.1093/geronb/gbab128.

Fung, Jason. 2016. *The Obesity Code: Unlocking the Secrets of Weight Loss*. Vancouver: Greystone Books.

Fung, Jason, and Jimmy Moore. 2016. *The Complete Guide to Fasting: Heal Your Body through Intermittent, Alternate-Day, and Extended Fasting*. Las Vegas: Victory Belt Publishing.

Gerber, Richard. 2001. *Vibrational Medicine: The #1 Handbook of Subtle Energy Therapies*. Rochester, VT: Bear & Company/Inner Traditions.

Goleman, Daniel. 2005. *Emotional Intelligence: Why It Can Matter More Than IQ*. New York: Random House.

Goleman, Daniel, and Richard J. Davidson. 2017. *Altered Traits: How Meditation Changes Your Mind, Brain, and Body*. New York: Avery/Penguin Random House.

Goleman, Daniel, and Richard J. Davidson. 2018. *The Science of Meditation: How to Change Your Brain, Mind and Body*. New York: Penguin Life.

Goleman, Daniel and Joel Gurin, eds. 1993. *Mind-Body Medicine: How to Use Your Mind for Better Health*. New York: Consumer Reports Books.

Goswami, Amit. 1995. *The Self-Aware Universe: How Consciousness Creates the Material World*. New York: Jeremy P. Tarcher/Putnam.

Goswami, Amit. 2004. *The Quantum Doctor: A Quantum Physicist Explains the Healing Power of Integral Medicine*. Charlottesville, VA: Hampton Roads.

Goswami, Amit. 2008. *Creative Evolution: A Physicist's Resolution Between Darwinism & Intelligent Design*. Wheaton, IL: Quest Books/Theosophical Publishing House.

Goswami, Amit. 2013. *Physics of the Soul: The Quantum Book of Living, Dying, Reincarnation, and Immortality*. Charlottesville, VA: Hampton Roads.

Goswami, Amit. 2013. *Quantum Creativity: Think Quantum, Be Creative*. New York: Hay House.

Goswami, Amit. 2017. *The Everything Answer Book: How Quantum Science

Explains Love, Death, and the Meaning of Life. Charlottesville, VA: Hampton Roads.

Goswami, Amit. 2022. *See the World as a Five Layered Cake*. Delhi, India: Blue Rose Publishers.

Goswami, Amit, and Valentina R. Onisor. 2019. *Quantum Spirituality: The Pursuit of Wholeness*. Delhi, India: Blue Rose Publishers.

Goswami, Amit, and Valentina R. Onisor. 2021. *The Quantum Brain: Understand, Rewire and Optimize Your Brain*. Eugene, OR: Luminare Press.

Goswami, Amit, and Sunita Pattani. 2022. *Quantum Psychology and the Science of Happiness*. Eugene, OR: Luminare Press.

Grof, Stan. 2019. *Realms of the Human Unconscious: Observations from LSD Research*. GautamBuddha Nagar, India: Souvenir Publishers.

Grof, Stan, and Christina Grof. 2010. *Holotropic Breathwork: A New Approach to Self-Exploration and Therapy*. SUNY Series in Transpersonal and Humanistic Psychology. Albany, NY: SUNY/Excelsior Editions.

Grossinger, Richard. 2001. *Planet Medicine: Origins*. Berkeley, CA: North Atlantic Books.

Grossman, Richard L. 1985. *The Other Medicines: An Invitation to Understanding Them & Using Them for Health & Healing*. New York: Doubleday.

Hahnemann, Samuel. (2008). *Organon of Homeopathic Medicine (1836)*. Whitefish, MT: Kessinger Publishing.

Hofstadter, Douglas R. 1999. *Gödel, Escher, Bach: An Eternal Golden Braid*. New York: Basic Books.

Howard, Benedick. 2005. "Cymatics: Highlights of a Meeting with Sir Peter Guy Manners and Benedick Howard." Interview by Benedick Howard in summer 1997, published on DreamWeaving International website. https://www.bibliotecapleyades.net/ciencia/ciencia_cymatics05.htm.

Joyce, James. 1914/2017. "A Painful Case." In *Dubliners*. London: Grant Richards Ltd. (first edition, 1914). Edinburgh: CrossReach Publications (paperback edition, 2017).

Kapleau, Roshi Philip. 1989. *The Three Pillars of Zen: Teaching, Practice, and Enlightenment*. New York: Anchor.

BIBLIOGRAPHY

Kent, J. T. (2002). *Repertory of the Homeopathic Materia Medica and a Word Index*. Uttar Pradesh, India: B. Jain Publishers.

Koestenbaum, Peter. 1974. *Managing Anxiety: The Power of Knowing Who You Are*. Hoboken, NJ: Prentice Hall.

Kragh, Helgi. 2012. *Niels Bohr and the Quantum Atom: The Bohr Model of Atomic Structure 1913–1925*. Oxford, UK: Oxford University Press.

Lad, Vasant. 1984. *Ayurveda: The Science of Self-Healing—A Practical Guide*. Santa Fe, NM: Lotus Press.

Le Fanu, James. 1999. *The Rise and Fall of Modern Medicine*. New York: Carrol & Graf.

Lipton, Bruce H. 2016. *The Biology of Belief: Unleashing the Power of Consciousness, Matter & Miracles*. New York: Hay House.

Macrae, Norman. 1992. *John von Newmann: The Scientific Genius Who Pioneered the Modern Computer, Game Theory, Nuclear Deterrence, and Much More*. New York: Pantheon Books.

Markolin, Caroline. 2007. *German New Medicine (GNM)—Dr. Hamer's Medical Paradigm*. Internet Archive. https://archive.org/details/MarkolinCarolineGermanNewMedicineDr.HamersMedicalParadigm20078P.

Maslow, Abraham H. 2013. *A Theory of Human Motivation*. Mansfield Centre, CT: Martino Publishing.

Mattson, Mark P. 2022. *The Intermittent Fasting Revolution: The Science of Optimizing Health and Enhancing Performance*. Cambridge, MA: MIT Press.

Mosley, Michael. 2020. *The Fast 800 Diet: Discover the Ideal Fasting Formula to Shed Pounds, Fight Disease, and Boost Your Overall Health*. New York: Atria/Simon & Schuster.

Moss, Richard. 1981. *The I That Is We: Awakening to Higher Energies through Unconditional Love*. Berkeley, CA: Celestial Arts.

Moss, Richard. 1987. *The Black Butterfly: An Invitation to Radical Aliveness*. Berkeley, CA: Celestial Arts.

Motz, Julie. 1998. *Energy Healer: An Energy Healer Reveals the Secrets of Using Your Body's Own Energy Medicine for Healing, Recovery, and Transformation*. New York: Bantam Books/Random House.

Page, Christine. 1992. *Frontiers of Health: How to Heal the Whole Person*. Saffron Walden, UK: C.W. Daniel.

Pagliaro, Gioacchino, N. Mandolisi, G. Parenti, L. Marconi, M. Galli, F. Sereci, and E. Augostini. 2017. "Human Bio-Photons Emission: An Observational Case Study of Emission of Energy Using a Tibetan Meditative Practice on an Individual." *BOAJ Physics* 2 (4): 1–9.

Pelletier, Kenneth R. 1977. *Mind as Healer, Mind as Slayer: A Holistic Approach to Preventing Stress Disorders*. New York: Delta.

Pelletier, Kenneth R. 1981. *Longevity: Fulfilling Our Biological Potential*. New York: Delacorte Press.

Penrose, Roger. 1996. *Shadows of the Mind: A Search for the Missing Science of Consciousness*. Oxford, UK: Oxford University Press.

Pert, Candace B. 1999. *Molecules of Emotion: The Science Behind Mind-Body Medicine*. New York: Simon & Schuster.

Pickles, Andrew, et al. (2016). "Parent-mediated social communication therapy for young children with autism (PACT): long-term follow-up of a randomized controlled trial." *The Lancet* 388 (10059): 2501–09.

Popper, Karl. Edited by Paul Arthur Schilpp. 1974/1988. *The Philosophy of Karl Popper*. 2 vols. LaSalle, IL: Open Court Publishing.

Radin, Dean, Nancy Lund, Masuro Emoto, and Takashige Kizu. 2008. "Effects of Distant Intention on Water Crystal Formation: A Triple-Blind Application." *Journal of Scientific Exploration* 22 (4): 481–93.

Rahe, Richard, and Thomas H. Holmes. (1967). "The Social Readjustment Rating Scale." *Journal of Psychosomatic Research* 11:213–18. https://www.mayfieldschools.org/Downloads/18%20Life%20Change%20and%20Stress2.pdf.

Ramachandran, V. S. 2012. *The Tell-Tale Brain: A Neuroscientist's Quest for What Makes Us Human*. New York: W. W. Norton.

Russell, Ronald. 2007. *The Journey of Robert Monroe: From Out-of-Body Explorer to Conscious Pioneer*. Charlottesville, VA: Hampton Roads.

Sacks, Oliver. 2008. *Musicophilia: Tales of Music and the Brain*. New York: Vintage/Random House.

Salovey, Peter, Marc A. Brackett, and John D. Mayer, eds. 2004. *Emotional Intelligence: Key Readings on the Mayer and Salovey Model*. Portchester,

BIBLIOGRAPHY

NY: Dude Publishing/National Professional Resources.

Sastri, V. V. Subrahmanya 2004. *Tridosha Theory: A Study on the Fundamental Principals of Ayurveda*. Kottakkal/Kerala, India: Radhakrishna Press.

Schlitz, Marilyn, and Tina Amorock, (with Marc S. Micozzi). 2004. *Consciousness and Healing: Integral Approaches to Mind-Body Medicine*. St. Louis, MO: Elsevier.

Searle, John R. 1994. *The Rediscovery of the Mind*. Cambridge, MA: MIT Press.

Sheldrake, Rupert. 1983. *A New Science of Life: The Hypothesis of Morphic Resonance*. Los Angeles: Tarcher.

Siegel, Bernie S. 1993. *Peace, Love & Healing: Bodymind Communication & the Path to Self-Healing—An Exploration*. New York: HarperPerennial.

Svoboda, Robert E., and Arnie Lade. 1995. *Tao and Dharma: Chinese Medicine and Ayurveda*. Twin Lakes, WI: Lotus Press.

The Quantum Activist. 2009. Produced and directed by Renee Slade and Ri Stewart, written by Ted Golder, featuring Amit Goswami. DVD. Portland, OR: Intention Media/BlueDot Productions.

Thompson, Jeffrey D. (1996/2010). "Sounds—Medicine for the New Millennium." In Dr. Thompson (articles). Center for Neuroacoustic Research. http://neuroacoustic.org/.

Tiller, William A. n.d. "Discovering the Power of Human Intention." In William A. Tiller/The Tiller Model, Papers and Interviews/Dr. Tiller's Work Explained. Tiller Foundation. https://www.tillerfoundation.org/_files/ugd/bbbea2_da7a72c09e154d529bfee0aacf225de8.pdf.

Tokyo Institute of Technology. 2012. Interview with Yoshinori Osumi. "Elucidating the Mechanism of Autophagy: It All Started with a Microscope— Autophagy, the Survival Strategy of Organisms." https://www.titech.ac.jp/english/public-relations/research/stories/ohsumi.

Ullman, Dana. 1987. *Homeopathy: Medicine for the 21st Century*. Berkeley, CA: North Atlantic Books.

Volk, Jeff. 2020. *Cymatics, Sound, Vibration and Creation—How Sound Animates Our World*. YouTube video. Ashland, OR: Rogue Valley Metaphysical Library. https://www.youtube.com/watch?v=lM3oHWUjsgo.

Wayne, Michael. 2005. *Quantum Integral Medicine: Towards a New Science of*

Healing and Human Potential. Saratoga Springs, NY: iThink Books.

Weil, Andrew. 1983. *Health and Healing: Understanding Conventional and Alternative Medicine.* Boston: Houghton Mifflin.

What the Bleep Do We Know? 2004. Feature film written, produced, and directed by William Arntz, Mark Vincente, and Betsy Chasse. Featuring Marlee Matlin, and others. Distributed by Gravitas Ventures, Cleveland, OH.

Willow, Katherine. 2019. *German New Medicine, Experiences in Practice: An introduction to the medical discoveries of Dr. Ryke Geerd Hamer.* Self-published.

Yanchi, Liu. 1988. *The Essential Book of Traditional Chinese Medicine—Volume I: Theory,* and *Volume 2: Clinical Practice.* Translated by Fang Tingyu and Chen Laidi. New York: Columbia University Press.

INDEX

5:20 diet, 204
16:8 diet, 204

Abusity, 273
Achterberg, Jeanne, 61
Acupressure, 113, 217
Acupuncture, 40, 111–16, 143
Adams, Patch, 84
Ader, Robert, 167
Advaitananda, 67, 68
Ageless body (immortality), 281–82
Aging, 255, 257–58
    See also Elderly people
Allopathy, 15
    See also Conventional medicine
Altered Traits (Goleman/Davidson), 38
Alternate nostril breathing, 207
Alternative deep inhaling, 273
Alzheimer's disease, 99, 164, 250–75, 266, 268
Ama, 140, 154, 259, 260, 267
Ankylosing spondylitis, 248–49
Anorexia, 176

Anterior cingulate cortex (ACC), 194
Anthropic principle, 71
Anxiety, 215–16
Apotemnophilia, 162
Archetypes, 277
Art therapy, 233
Arthritis, 117, 176
Aspect, Alain, 22
Asthi, 128
Astringent and pungent tastes, 261
Attention, 78, 81, 183
    See also Inattention
Attention deficit disorder, 225
Attention deficit hyperactive disorder (ADHD), 171
Augustine, Saint, 249
Augustus, Caesar, 97
Aurobindo, Sri, 19
Austin, James, 208
Autism, 171
Autophagy, 205
Avogadro's law of chemistry, 118
Awakening of Intelligence, The (Goswami/Onisor), 281

Awareness, 265
Awareness meditation, 208
Ayurveda
   bowel movements, 164
   cleansing the system, 154
   common sense, 146
   defined, 72
   diagnosing disease by reading pulse, 114, 116
   dosha imbalances, 136–37
   five elements theory, 127, 140
   fundamental assumption, 125
   general principles about vital liturgical fields, 138
   heart disease, 131–32
   herbal medicines, 41
   heterogeneity, 262
   individualized treatments, 139
   loss of appetite, 261
   nadi testing, 116
   nadis, 111f
   nonmaterial medicine system, 16
   reincarnation, 130
   six tastes, 200
   tejas and pitta, 139
   traditional Indian medicine, 16
   treating vital components of disease, 46
   unbalanced application of gunas, 170
   vata imbalances, 146
   yoga, 149–50

Badrasana, 153
Barasch, Marc, 234–35
Bardo, 253
Bee test, 66
Beer belly, 262, 263
Benson, Herbert, 225
Bereavement, 189
Berra, Yogi, 228
Bhakti yoga, 226
Big pharma, 95–96, 274–75
Bioelectric body, 1–2
Biology of Belief, The (Lipton), 19
Black Butterfly, The (Moss), 235
Black Monday syndrome, 166
Blake, Carl, 273
Bliss body, 38, 229–30
Blocked chakra, 164, 218–21
Bodies of human being. *See* Five bodies of the human being
Body types, 124–25
Body's wisdom, 60, 259
Bohr, Niels, 63f
Booth-Kewley, Stephanie, 179
Brain
   anterior cingulate cortex (ACC), 194
   connected to organs of physical body, 44
   hypothalamus, 264
   memory-making capacity, 5
   neocortex, 187
   neuropeptides, 168
   parietal lobe, 269
   prefrontal cortex, 222–23
   response to hormone activity, 265
   tangled hierarchy, 53–58
Breast cancer, 181–91
balancing heart and navel chakra functioning, 191
   Herring's law, 120
   Jolie, Angelina, 185
   Kirlian photography, 189–90

INDEX

love, 185
mind-body disease, 189
why do cells go rogue?, 191
Breathing practices, 206–7
  See also Pranayama
Broken leg, 79–80
Brow chakra
  aging, 266–69
  Alzheimer's disease, 164
  associated organs, 33*f*
  awakening, 9
  concentrating on something intellectual, 156
  concentration/awareness meditation, 208
  diseases, 162
  vital energy, 34
Buddha, 55, 92–93
Buddhi, 280
Bully phenomenon, 134
Burnout, 91
Byrd, Randolph, 61

Cancer
  breast. *See* Breast cancer
  cause, 44
  chakra disease, 161
  creative visualization, 234, 235
  disease of not living enough, 100
  heart chakra, 164
  immune system malfunction, 33, 175
  love, 176, 183
  spontaneous healing, 236
  sudden insight, 235–36
Capturing the Uncaught Mind (tratakam), 154

Cardiovascular system, 260
Causal body, 42
Chakra, 32
  See also Chakra medicine
Chakra medicine
  activation of chakras, 163
  blocking/unblocking of chakras, 164, 218–21
  brain-mind takeover of chakras, 166–68
  chakra, defined, 32
  concomitant chakra psychology, 163
  movement of energy from one chakra to another, 163
  overview, 33*f*, 162
  vitalizing chakras, 163
  See also individual chakras
Chanting, 208
Chemical imbalance theory, 274–75
Chi, 4
  See also Prana
Chi gong, 265
Chinese medicine. *See* Traditional Chinese Medicine
Cholesterol, 266
Chopra, Deepak, 12, 16, 63, 125, 141, 184, 235–36
Christian Science, 238
Chronic disease, 139–40
Chronic fatigue syndrome, 177
Circularity, 54, 57*f*
Cleansing the system, 154
  See also Panchakarma
Collapsing possibility waves, 41, 42*f*, 132, 165, 190
Common cold, 140

Competitiveness, 174, 175
Complete Guide to Fasting (Fung/Moore), 204
Compromising, 99
Computers, symbol-processing machines, 35
Concentration meditation, 208, 222, 223, 225
Conditioning, 59, 60
Confucius, 229
Congruence, 279
Consciousness
  actualizing both perception and memory apparatuses, 56
  beauty and wholeness, 77
  collapse of waves of possibility, 165
  epigenetic programs of instruction, 10
  expansion of, 77, 244
  genetic disposition, 186
  ground of being, 278
  importance, 1, 5
  Jung (making the unconscious conscious), 71
  little/big expansions, 77
  liturgical fields, 107
  mediating between vital and physical bodies, 41, 42*f*
  mental software, 30
  morphogenetic fields, 31
  persevering with surrender, 246
  separate from other actualized objects, 54
  splitting itself into two parts, 56
  traumatic memory, 217
  vital-physical connection, 191
Constipation, 261

Conventional medicine
  disease-centered mindset, 3, 7, 13, 67, 93
  emergency medicine, 183
  evidence-based medicine, 22
  five metaphysical shortcomings, 28–29
  genes, 123
  lacking comprehensive underlying theory, 22
  looking at the problem from wrong end, 67
Corona virus, 270, 272
Cousins, Norman, 248
Covid 19 (corona virus), 270–74
Creative Evolution (Goswami), 19
Creative healing, 33
Creative Integrative Medicine (Drouin), 12
Creative process, 79–80, 236–37, 247
"Creative sleep," 230
Creative visualization, 234–35
Creativity
  creative qualities and quality of conditioning, 170
  differentiating between various types, 129
  fundamental. *See* Fundamental creativity
  purity of intention, 239–40
  self-healing, 245
  situational. *See* Situational creativity
  supramental intelligence, 280
  vital, 3, 33
Crown chakra
  aging and cognitive decline, 269

INDEX

associated feelings, 158f, 160
associated organs, 33f
diseases, 162
vital energy, 34
Cymatics, 86

Davidson, Richard, 38, 222
de Chardin, Teilhard, 19, 71
Death, 256, 278
Deep meditation, 247–49
Dementia, 99, 100, 267
    See also Alzheimer's disease
Dependent coarising, 58, 59
Depression, 45, 274–75
Descartes, Rene, 51
Dharma, 195, 228–29
Dhatus, 128, 133
Diabetes, 66–67
    See also Type II diabetes
Dilbert (comic strip), 221
Discount, 95
Disease
    absence of health, 75
    all five bodies of human being, 46–47
    breaking laws of science and consciousness, 74
    incongruence, 279
    objective malfunctioning of organism, 43
    reminder to change our ways, 36
    yin-yang imbalance, 137
Disease-prone personality, 177–79
Distance healing, 61
Do-be-do-be-do
    alternating dancing or Tai chi with relaxation of healing meditation, 234

art therapy, 233
creative healing, 232–33
creativity, 170
defined, 129
fasting, 202
fundamental creativity, 245–46
heart chakra energy block, 238–39
nourishment for supplemental level, 227
pranayama, 273–74
quantum creativity, 245
sattvic and rajasic people, 226
vital energy, 255
yoga asana practice, 259
Do-do-do, 145, 147, 153, 171, 259, 273
Doshas
    defined, 128, 135
    imbalances, 16, 143, 225
    kapha. *See* Kapha
    mind-brain, 170–72, 178
    pitta. *See* Pitta
    rules for determining your dosha, 141–42
    vata. *See* Vata
Dossey, Larry, 12, 192
Downward causation, 5, 30, 49, 56, 60–61, 64, 233
Dowsing, 120
Drawing Hands (Escher), 56, 57f
Drouin, Paul, 12
Dynamization, 16

Eating, 83
Eddy, Mary Baker, 238
EFT. *See* Emotional freedom technique (EFT)

Ego, 5, 52, 59–60
Ego-inflation, doctor, joke, 50
Eigen, Manfred, 19
Elderly people
  brain's response to hormone activity, 265
  brow chakra, 266
  Covid 19 (corona virus), 270
  death, 256
  elimination system, 260–61
  endocrine system, 264–66
  geriatric syndromes, 269
  heart-chakra organs, 263
  influenza, 270
  materialist approach to gerontology, 252
  metabolism and visceral fat, 261–63
  motivation is key to healthy aging, 252–53
  navel chakra organs, 261–63
  organ function deterioration, 258–60
  quality of life, 251, 256
  tasks of quantum gerontology, 253–54
  theory of aging, 255, 257–58
Emotional awareness, 210–11
Emotional freedom technique (EFT), 217
Emotional intelligence, 194, 209–10, 211
Emotional Intelligence (Goleman), 209
Emotional memory, 216–18
Emotional patterns, 211, 212–14
Emotional personality patterns, 214–16
Emotional stress, 36, 165–66
Emotions
  expressing, 172–75
  feeling component, 155
  negative, 194
  prana, 109
  primordial emotional level, 208–9
  suppressing, 175–77
Emoto, Masaru, 4–5
Empathy, 59, 62, 62f, 91, 92, 109
Endorphins, 168–69
Enlightenment, 47–48
Environmental effect, 82
Epictetus, 192
Escher's hand, 56, 57f
Evidence-based medicine, 22, 251
Evo-devo, 77
Expressing emotions, 172–75

Fast yoga, 259
Fasting, 202–4
Fear, 106, 180, 215
Feelings, 46, 180
Fibromyalgia, 177
Five bodies of the human being, 10, 11f, 42
Five elements theory, 127, 128, 140
Flow experience, 227
Flow meditation, 227
Flu, 270
Food. *See* Nutrition
Forced vibration, 76
Forest Gump (film), 171
Frawley, David, 125, 141
Free will, 60
Freidman, Howard S., 179
Freud, Sigmund, 76

INDEX

Freund, Alexandra M., 252
Frontiers of Health: How to Heal the Whole Person (Page), 160, 218
Frustration, 175
Fundamental creativity
    bliss body, 229
    defined, 37
    healing, 232–37
    perseverance, 245
    quantum leap, 196, 231, 239
    rajas, 226
    regeneration of stem cells, 261
    sattva, 170
    soul-making, 243
    tejas, 130, 131, 133, 134, 147
    vital potentiality, 135
Fung, Jason, 203, 204

Gandhi, Mahatma, 90
Genes, 123
Genetic disposition, 186
Geriatric syndromes, 269
Gerontology. *See* Elderly people
God, 64, 243, 244
Gödel's incompleteness theorem, 35
Goedel, Escher, Bach (Hofstadter), 54
Goleman, Daniel, 38, 209, 222
Grof, Stan, 38, 253
Gross body, 42
Groundhog Day (film), 74
Guided imagery, 219–20
Guna (gunas), 125, 132–33, 169–70, 225

Hahnemann, Samuel, 117
Hamer, Ryke Geerd, 179–80
Happiness, 58, 222–23, 244, 277
    See also Unhappiness
Hara, 188
Hardware-software connection, 10, 30, 32*f*, 72, 272
Hatha yoga, 217, 221, 227
Hayflick, Leonard, 182, 257
Hayflick effect, 257, 282
Headache, 176
Healer, 89–101
    burnout, 91
    empathy, 92
    healing vs. curing pain, 93–97
    how to become a healer, 101
    initial talk with patient, 101
    principle of reflection, 89, 91
    principle of resonance, 89
    quantum worldview, 99
    self-healing, 89, 92
    self-transformation, 96
    walking the talk, 92, 101
Healing Path, The (Barasch), 234–35
Healing yourself, 89
    See also Self-healing
Health, 75, 85
Health and Healing (Weil), 20
Health insurance, 98
Heart chakra
    associated feelings, 158*f*, 159
    associated organs, 33*f*
    awakening, 9
    balancing heart and navel chakra functioning, 191
    blocked chakras, 218–19
    breast cancer, 181–91
    cancer, 164
    diseases, 161
    elderly people, 263

energy block, 238–39
laughing meditation, 208
love, 181
vital energy, 34
Heart disease, 131–32
Heart Math Institute, 6
Hedge, B. Monappa, 237
Heisenberg's uncertainty principle, 112
Herring's law, 120
Heterogeneity, 262
High blood pressure, 260
Higher self, 58
Hippocrates, 202
Hofstadter, Doug, 54
Holistic health, 252
Holotropy, 253, 254, 255, 275, 277
Homeo-stenosis, 258, 259
Homeopathy, 15–16, 17, 28, 116–20, 138
Hostility, 174, 175, 219
Human development, 253
Hunger and fullness signals, 201
Hylotropy, 253
Hyperactivity
   attention deficit disorder, 224–25
   do-do-do lifestyle, 171
   dominant rajasic dosha, 172
   mind-brain doshas, 173
   slowing down, 224
Hypertension, 260
Hypothalamus, 264
Hypothyroidism, 264

"I" experience, 51–52, 58, 59
Ignorance, 72
Illness, 43, 74
Immortality, 281–82
Immune inflammation theory of psychosis, 275
Immune system, 167, 187, 188, 271
Inattention, 78–79
   See also Attention
Incongruence, 279
Incubation, 80
Indian medicine. *See* Ayurveda
Individuality, 36
Inertia, 132, 267
   See also Ojas
Inflammation, 266–67
Influenza, 270
Information and social media, 221–22, 268
Inner self, 58
Intellectualism, 223
Interaction dualism, 10
Internal hygiene, 13, 154
   See also Panchakarma
Internet, 221–22
Intuition, 9, 30, 58
Iron-man syndrome, 263
Irritability, 173, 174
Ishwara Pranidhana, 247

Jing, 265
Jnana yoga, 226
Jolie, Angelina, 185
Journal, 88, 210
Joyce, James, 223–25
Juicy physicality, 223
Jung, Carl, 71, 77, 219

Kapalavati, 208
Kapha, 126, 133, 135
   diseases caused by congestion, 131

INDEX

earth and water, 127
inner fire (agni) tends to run low, 150
lifestyle remedies, 148–49
stalky and robust, 134
yoga, 150–51
Kapleau, Roshi Philip, 196
Keating, Thomas, 213
Keats, John, 276
Kharma yoga, 226
King-minister story, 193
Kirlian photography, 4, 189–90
Koestenbaum, Peter, 215
Krishna, 65
Kumbhaka, 274
Kundalini, 255
Kundalini awakening, 255, 265
Kung-yen Vow, 91

Lack of appetite, 136
Lad, Vasant, 141
Lade, Arnie, 143
Laughing meditation, 208, 220
Lawrence, Brother, 227–28
LCU. *See* Life change unit (LCU)
Less-is-more axiom, 118, 119
Lethargic vitality, 260
Liar's sentence, 54, 55
Life change unit (LCU), 166
Like-cures-like medicine, 117, 118
Lipton, Bruce, 19
Little Prince, The (de Saint-Exupéry), 181–82
Liturgical fields, 31, 33, 45, 107, 138, 156, 182–83
Liver, stomach, and meridians, 184–85
Longevity, 251

Loss of appetite, 261
Love
cancer, 176, 183
coherence, 190
family, 139
heart chakra, 181
immune system malfunction, 175, 189
immune system stressors, 168
mental stress, 186
other-love, 139, 140
preventive measure, 186
romantic, 135, 187
self-love, 139, 140
suspension of immune system, 190

Magritte, Rene, 222
Maharshi, Ramana, 48
Maitreyi, 281
Majja, 128
Male-female differences, 188, 191
Mamsa, 128
Managing Anxiety (Koestenbaum), 215
Manifestation, 236–37
Manipura asanas, 150
Manners, Peter Guy, 86
Mantra chanting, 86, 87
Markolin, Caroline, 180
Maslow, Abraham, 275
Material monism, 4, 22, 95
Materialist worldview, 27, 95, 97
Mattson, Mark, 203, 204
Meaning and Medicine (Dossey), 192
Meats, 200–201
Meda, 128

Meditation, 194–95, 223–25
    awareness, 208, 223
    concentration, 208, 222, 223, 225
    deep, 247–49
    flow, 227
    happiness, 222–23
    laughing, 208, 220
    mental agitation, 153
    peace, 220
    relaxation response, 225
    sacred, 206
Meditation on peace, 220
Memento mori, 97
Mental body, 42
Mental environment, 44
Mental hygiene, 221, 229
Mental pollution, 221
Mentalization, 194–96
Mentalization of feelings, 46, 180
Meridians, 110, 111*f*, 112–14, 115*f*, 185
Metabolic syndrome, 262
Midbrain chakra, 264–66
Midlife transition, 253
Mind-body medicine, 15, 47, 165
Mind-brain dosha, 170–72, 178
Molecules of Emotion (Pert), 168
Monroe, Robert, 87
Moore, Jimmy, 204
Morphogenetic fields, 31, 157
    See also Liturgical fields
Mosley, Michael, 204
Moss, Richard, 223, 235
Mother Teresa effect, 168
Motivation, 252–53
Motz, Julie, 217
Muladhara asanas, 153

Muscle testing, 113
Music, 85–87
My Fair Lady (film), 221

Nadi testing, 116
Nadis, 110, 111*f*
Namaste greeting, 162
Nan Lu, 191
Nasruddin, Mulla, 170–71
Nature vs. nurture, 130
Naturopathy, 138
Navel chakra
    associated feelings, 158*f*, 159
    associated organs, 33*f*
    awakening, 9
    balancing heart and navel chakra functioning, 191
    blocked chakras, 218–19
    cognition apparatus, 188
    diseases, 161
    elderly people, 261–63
    laughing meditation, 208
    type II diabetes, 164
Near-death experiences, 278–79
Negative emotions, 194
Negative meaning, 45
Negative resonance, 78–80, 85
Neo-Darwinism, 19, 20
Neocortex, 187
Neuropeptides, 168
Nonlocality, 8, 61, 91, 219
Nutrition, 199–205
    5:20 diet, 204
    16:8 diet, 204
    autophagy, 205
    fasting, 202–4
    feeling of expansiveness, 201
    hunger and fullness signals, 201

INDEX

meats, 200–201
occasional dalliance, 200
six tastes, 200
soul food, 222

Obesity, 148, 263
Obesity Code: Unlocking the Secrets of Weight Loss, The (Fung), 204
Observer effect, 9, 52, 53
Oceanic feelings, 77
Of Sound Mind & Body: Music & Vibrational Healing (Sheldrake), 86
Ojas
    abdominal fat, 262
    child development, 148
    chronic disease, 128
    formative years, 130
    inertia, 132, 267
    obesity, 148
    organ function, 133
    romantic love, 135
    seasons, 144
    stalky and robust, 134
Older people. *See* Elderly people
Oneness, 243
Opening, 255
Other-love, 139, 140, 191

P-organ, 32*f*
Page, Christine, 160, 161, 218
Pagliario, Gioacchino, 5
Pain, 93, 100, 177
"Painful Case, A" (Joyce), 223
Panchakarma, 136, 154, 259, 261
Paracelsus, 65
Parasympathetic nervous system, 151, 173, 207
Parietal lobe, 269
Parre, Jacques, 65
Particles, 8
Patanjali, 46, 226, 247
Pattani, Sunita, 277
Peace, Love & Healing (Siegel), 280
Penrose, Roger, 35
Peptic ulcer, 174
Perseverance, 245, 246
Personal God, 243, 244
Personality development, 213
Perspiration, 264
Pert, Candace, 168
Pharmaceutical industry (big pharma), 95–96, 274–75
Physical body, 42
Physical environment, 44
Physics of the Soul (Goswami), 130
Physiology, 3, 6
Pitta, 127, 134, 135
    heart chakra and navel chakra organ disease, 135
    lifestyle remedies, 147–48
    liquid and gas, 127
    tejas, 127, 147
    yoga, 151–52
Pituitary gland, 264
Placebo cure (placebo effect), 82, 117, 232, 237
Plaisir, 212
Popper, Karl, 19
Positive attitude (king-minister story), 193
Positive emotional personality patterns, 214–16
Positive intentions and thoughts, 79
Positive resonance, 80
Prakriti, 16, 69, 130, 137, 149, 150

Prana
　defined, 108
　emotions, 109
　exercise for understanding how prana works, 162–63
　pranayama, 207
　sacred meditation, 206
　vital energy, 4
　Western culture, 27
Pranayama, 137, 206–7, 221, 227, 274
Prefrontal cortex, 222–23
Preventive medicine, 75
Primordial emotional level, 208–9
Principle of reflection, 89, 91
Promissory materialism, 19
Psycho-neuro-endocrinology, 168–69
Psycho-neuro-immuno-gastro-intestinology, 187
Psycho-neuro-immunology, 166–68
Psychoanalysis, 216–17
Psychodynamics, 217
Purity of intention, 239–40

Quality of life, 186, 251
Quantum activism, 185
Quantum biology, 23
Quantum creativity, 245
　See also Creativity
Quantum Doctor, The (Goswami)
　author's limited understanding of health issues, 7
　fMRI, 5
　homeopathy, 117
　Kirlian photography, 4
　quantum healing, 231

Quantum entities, 211
Quantum entrepreneurship, 254
Quantum healing, 68, 231
Quantum Healing (Chopra), 235–36
Quantum health management, 14
Quantum integrative medicine
　basic quantum principles, 60–61
　crowning achievement, 30
　goal, 48
　integrative science of experience, 13
　key concepts, 48–49, 74
　maintaining health of all five of our bodies, 43
　two aspects, 20
　weakly objective and therefore scientific, 50
Quantum leap, 63, 63f, 231, 239
Quantum metaphysics, 8
Quantum physics
　consciousness, 5
　objects, 8
　physics of possibility, 270
　subject/self, 52–53
　suppressing emotions, 176–77
　whole being, 41
Quantum Psychology and the Science of Happiness (Goswami/Pattani), 214, 277
Quantum reality, 70
Quantum self, 55, 58, 73, 226
Quantum thinking, 49
Quantum worldview, 1, 20, 21, 59, 100, 186
Quantum yoga, 199, 238–39, 262
　See also Yoga

INDEX

Radiant forehead (kapalavti), 208
Radin, Dean, 5
Rahe, Richard, 166
Raja yoga, 226
Rajas, 169–72, 225, 226
Rakta, 128
Ramachandran, V. S., 162
Ramakrishna, 48
Rasa, 128
Rasayana, 261
Rediscovery of the Mind, The (Searle), 29
Regeneration, 105, 257, 261
Reiki, 109, 137
Reincarnation, 40, 130, 171, 256, 278–79
Reincarnational heritage, 132
Relaxation response, 38
Relaxation Response, The (Benson), 225
Resilience, 246
Resonance, 76–88
    Adams, Patch, 84
    applying principle of resonance in practice, 83, 84, 89
    frequency and sound of healing, 85–87
    frequency matching, 76
    main, 81
    negative, 78–80, 85
    positive, 80
    resonating on many levels at same time, 81
    sympathetic, 86
Rest, 271, 272
Rolfing, 217
Romantic love, 135, 187
    See also Love

Root chakra
    associated feelings, 158, 158*f*
    associated organs, 33*f*
    blocked chakras, 218
    diseases, 161
    feelings of fear or security, 133
    walking barefoot, 208

Sacks, Oliver, 37
Sacred meditation, 206
Salovey, Peter, 209
Samadi, 58
Sastri, V. V. Subrahmanya, 129
Sattva, 169, 170, 225, 226, 277
Scientist, 70
Searle, John, 35
Seasons, 144
Self, 58, 190
Self-Aware Universe, The (Goswami), 9, 53
Self-healing, 49, 64, 89, 91, 245, 248–49
Self-identity, 39, 54, 57*f*, 162, 184, 269
Self-love, 9, 139, 140, 191
Self-transformation, 96
Self-worth, 9, 134
Seven Is, 21, 214
Sex chakra
    associated feelings, 158*f*, 159
    associated organs, 33*f*
    blocked chakras, 218–19
    diseases, 161
    unfulfilled lust, 175
    vital energy when feeling amorous, 156
Sheldrake, Rupert, 31, 86, 157
Shen, 265

Shukra, 128
Siegel, Bernie, 280
Singing, chanting, 208
Sisyphus, 66
Situational creativity
   adjusting organ software, 40
   arthritis, 117
   body mechanisms, 258
   child/adult development, 130
   defined, 37
   healing powers, 237
   physical body homeostasis, 145
   rajas, 170
   throat chakra imbalance, 220
   vayu, 132, 135
   visualization, 220
Sivananda, Swami, 219
Six tastes, 200, 261
Slow yoga, 259
Slowing down, 224
Software-hardware connection, 10, 30, 32f, 72, 74, 272
Somatoparaphrenia, 162
Sonar facial lifting, 86
Sood, Sanjeev, 131
Soul, 37, 38, 276
Soul food, 222
Soul-making, 37–38, 73, 216, 243, 277
Sound and music, 85–87
Spicy food, 136, 144, 148
Spiritual enlightenment, 47–48
Spiritual healing, 7, 16, 17, 41
Spontaneous healing, 11, 63
States experienced during typical day, 199
Stomach ulcer, 166
Stress, 36, 165–66

Stressor, 165
Subject-object polarity, 53
Subtle body, 42
Subtle energy, 28
Sun salutations, 150
Suppression of emotions, 175–77
Supramental body, 37, 42, 227
Supramental healing, 47
Supramental intelligence
   cellular level, 282
   congruence, 279–80
   generally, 280–81
Surya namaskara, 150, 151
Svoboda, Robert E., 143
Sympathetic nervous system, 151, 173
Sympathetic resonance, 86

Taffet, G. E., 258
Tagore, Rabindranath, 145
Tai chi, 216, 221, 234
Tamas, 169–71, 225, 226
Tangled hierarchy, 53, 54, 58, 59, 91
Tantra, 255
Tao and Dharma: Chinese Medicine and Ayurveda (Svoboda/Lade), 143
Tastes, six, 200
Tejas
   aging, 259
   astringent and pungent tastes, 261
   chronic disease, 128
   digestive system, 147
   first appears at age of six, 130
   fundamental creativity, 130, 131, 133, 134, 147

INDEX

heart chakra and navel chakra
organ disease, 135
higher functional level, 134
lack of appetite, 136
pitta, 127, 147
romantic love, 135
soul-making, 277
spicy food, 136, 144, 148
vital creativity, 128
yoga, 263
Tell-Tale Brain, The
(Ramachandran), 162
Telomere, 257
Therapeutic tapping, 217
Third eye, 156, 160, 220
Three Pillars of Zen, The (Kapleau), 196
Throat chakra
associated feelings, 158f, 159–60
associated organs, 33f
diseases, 162
imbalance of vital energy, 220
singing, chanting, 208
vital energy, 34
Tibetan bowls, 87
Tiller, William, 120
Touch therapy, 217
Traditional Chinese Medicine
acupuncture, 15, 111–16
body types, 124–25
diagnosing disease by reading pulse, 114
five elements theory, 127, 140
general principles about vital liturgical fields, 138
herbal medicine, 15
individualized treatments, 139

meridians, 110, 111f, 112–14, 115f
Taoism, 124
treating vital components of disease, 46
yin and yang. *See* Yin and yang
Transpersonal self, 58
Tratakam (Capturing the Uncaught Mind), 154
Tridosha Theory (Sastri), 129
Trikonasana, 150
Type II diabetes, 121, 164, 203, 261, 262, 264

Ulcer, 174
Unhappiness, 72, 222
See also Happiness
Upward causation, 30

V-organ, 32f
Vata, 126–27
extremely active thinkers, 153
gas and emptiness or ether, 127
lifestyle remedies, 145–47
vayu, 127, 258
yoga, 153–54
Vayu, 132–33
adult years, 130
aging, 258
ama, 267
body's wisdom, 259
chronic disease, 128
coronary blockage, 174
creativity, 129
diseases caused by congestion, 131
dynamism, 133
hardening of the arteries, 260

romantic love, 135
seasons, 144
situational creativity, 132, 135
vata, 127, 258
yoga, 263
Viagra sex, 156
Vibrational medicine, 28, 34, 86
Vibrational Medicine (Gerber), 28
Victimhood and helplessness, 85
Vikriti, 128
Visceral fat, 262
Visualization, 219–20, 234–35, 245–46
Vital body, 31, 42, 44, 109
Vital creativity, 3, 33, 265
Vital energy, 4, 27–28, 34, 105, 108, 112, 255
  See also Prana
Vital energy exercises, 206–8
Vital software, 77
Volk, Jeff, 86
von Newmann, John, 9, 52, 53

Walking your talk, 91
Waves, 8
Weil, Andrew, 20, 48
Wholeness, 14, 47, 48, 59, 67, 91
Wolf, Fred Alan, 237
World as a Five-Layered Cake, The (Goswami), 55

Yajnabalkya, 281
Yin and yang
  acupuncture, 40
  balancing yin and yang, 39, 40
  body types, 124
  chi's two complementary aspects, 110, 111, 124
  classifying organs, 127
  common cold, 140
  defined, 110
  inflammation, 267
  organ function, 113, 133
  well-being, 205
Yoga
  awakening of midbrain chakra, 265
  Ayurveda, 149–50
  bhakti, 226
  developing best practice for your body type, 149–50
  fast, 259
  hatha, 217, 221, 227
  integration, 199
  jnana, 226
  kapha-dominant people, 150–51
  kharma, 226
  letting go of our tensions, 216
  metabolic syndrome, 262
  pitta-dominant people, 151–52
  quantum, 199, 238–39
  raja, 226
  slow, 259
  tejas, 263
  vayu, 263
  vita-dominant people, 153–54
  Western thought, 226–27
Young people, 69

Zen, 196

ABOUT THE AUTHORS

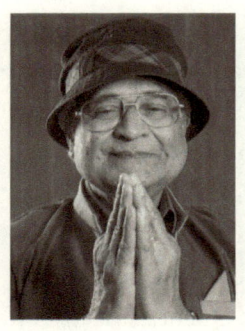

Dr. Amit Goswami is a retired professor in the physics department of the University of Oregon and a renowned pioneer of the new paradigm of quantum science based on the primacy of consciousness. He has written several groundbreaking books on research on quantum science and consciousness, including *The Self-Aware Universe, The Quantum Brain,* and *Quantum Spirituality* (with Valentina R. Onisor); and *The Quantum Doctor, Physics of the Soul, Quantum Creativity,* and *The Everything Answer Book.*

In 2009, Amit founded the Quantum Activism movement, which is now gaining ground in North America, South America, Europe, and India. In 2019, he and his cofounders established Quantum Activism Vishwalayam, operating as the department of Quantum Science at the University of Technology in Jaipur, India; the organization has also developed Master's and Ph.D. degrees in an international program of transformative education called the Quantum Science of Health, Prosperity, and Happiness.

Amit is featured in the film *What the Bleep Do We Know?* and the documentaries *The Dalai Lama Renaissance* and *The Quantum Activist.* He is also a spiritual practitioner who calls himself a "quantum activist in search of Wholeness."

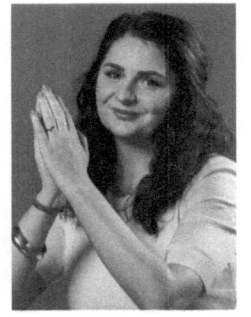**Valentina R. Onisor, M.D.,** is a practicing physician and a pioneer of quantum integrative medicine specializing in family medicine. She integrates conventional medicine with various systems of alternative medicine (including acupuncture, Ayurveda, naturopathy, and aromatherapy).

Committed to consciousness awakening-related sciences for over two decades, Valentina is also a yoga and meditation teacher (Sivananda Vedanta Forest Academy; Yoga Alliance; Universal Consciousness Ambassador, Center for the Study of Extraterrestrial Intelligence). Together with Dr. Amit Goswami, she has developed the transformative practice of Quantum Yoga, which integrates quantum science with traditional spiritual practices (yoga, qi gong, meditation, esoteric Christianity, and Tibetan Buddhism).

As a leader in transformational education, Valentina serves as a teacher and dean of students at Quantum Activism Vishwalayam, India, which she cofounded. She is a lecturer at Quantum Academy in Brazil and an acting consultant for the Center for Quantum Activism in Eugene, Oregon. Valentina is currently offering a number of courses and workshops oriented towards healing and spiritual transformation.

She is a coauthor (along with Dr. Amit Goswami) of the books *Quantum Spirituality* and *The Quantum Brain* and is currently working on additional books with Dr. Goswami on the awakening of intelligence, the return of the archetypes, and the quantum science of love and relationships.

www.ingramcontent.com/pod-product-compliance
Lightning Source LLC
Chambersburg PA
CBHW030135170426
43199CB00008B/69